The Modern Management
of
Mental Handicap

A Manual of Practice

EDITED BY

G. B. Simon

Director
The British Institute of Mental Handicap

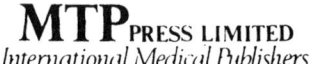

MTP PRESS LIMITED
International Medical Publishers

Published by
MTP Press Limited
Falcon House
Lancaster, England

Copyright © 1980 The British Institute of Mental Handicap

softcover reprint of the hardcover 1st edition 1980

British Library Cataloguing in Publication Data

The modern management of mental handicap.
  1. Mentally handicapped – Care and treatment
I. Simon, G.B.
  362.3   HV3004

ISBN 978-94-011-7202-8   ISBN 978-94-011-7200-4 (eBook)
DOI 10.1007/978-94-011-7200-4

Phototypesetting by Swiftpages Limited, Liverpool

REDWOOD BURN LIMITED
Trowbridge and Esher

CONTENTS

LIST OF CONTRIBUTORS

R. S. BLUGLASS
Professor of Forensic Psychiatry
University of Birmingham

J. A. CORBETT
Consultant Physician
Hilda Lewis House
The Bethlem Royal Hospital
Shirley, Croydon

V. A. COWIE
Consultant Psychiatrist
Queen Mary's Hospital for
Children
Carshalton

M. A. CRAFT
Personal Social Worker
Bryn-y-Neuadd Hospital
Llanfairfechan, Gwynedd

M. J. CRAFT
Consultant Psychiatrist
Bryn-y-Neuadd Hospital
Llanfairfechan, Gwynedd

N. B. CRAWFORD
Headmaster
Mary Elliot School
Walsall

J. JANCAR
Consultant Psychiatrist
Stoke Park Hospital
Stapleton, Bristol

E. JONES
Consultant Psychiatrist
Lea Castle Hospital
Wolverley, Kidderminster

MRS L. MARKS
Parent

P. MITTLER
Director
Hester Adrian Research Centre for
the Study of Learning Processes
in the Mentally Handicapped
and Professor of Special
Education
University of Manchester

v

M. PHILLIPS
Associate Director
Development Team for Mentally
Handicapped

D. M. RICKS
Consultant Psychiatrist
The Children's Department
Harperbury Hospital
Shenley, Radlett

B. I. SACKS
Consultant Psychiatrist
Enfield District Hospital
and Royal Free Hospital,
Hampstead

G. B. SIMON
Consultant Psychiatrist
Lea Castle Hospital
Kidderminster

J.C.N. TIBBITS
Medical Assistant
Lea Castle Hospital
Wolverley, Kidderminster

M. WALKER
Senior Speech Therapist
Botleys Park Hospital
Chertsey
Project Co-ordinator
Makaton Vocabulary Develop-
    ment Project
Farnborough

C. WILLIAMS
Principal Clinical Psychologist
Royal Western Counties Hospital
Starcross
Exeter

PREFACE

The aim of this book is to provide parents, staff and others involved with mentally handicapped children and adults with up-to-date basic information and advice in their management.

Methods of care, treatment and management of a heterogeneous group of people such as the mentally handicapped must of necessity include many disciplines if they are to be given an adequate service. This book is an attempt to bring the knowledge and experience of many people together. The size of the book could have been increased to include more detail on other aspects of the subject but this might easily have diminished its value as a convenient reference to as wide a readership as possible, both professional and non-professional.

The contents deal essentially with the needs of the severely mentally handicapped and should have an application in most parts of the world. Much of the information and advice on services, and on treatment and management, is based on the experience of specialists working in the United Kingdom, this now being standard practice in most parts of the world.

All the contributors have experienced direct involvement with the mentally handicapped, and have been chosen because of their specialized knowledge of particular aspects of the subject. To meet the needs of this wide readership, the authors have provided explanations which will enable readers to gain an understanding of the subject without previous related knowledge. Despite the intentional simplification the subject has been covered in the widest sense, and where more detail was not felt to be appropriate in this book, the lists of references and further reading suggested should provide further information.

Mental handicap, and severe mental handicap in particular, are crippling states in a world where increasingly only the fittest can achieve independent survival. Those less able tend to go under. Throughout this book the need for early assessment, treatment and training is stressed; this will not cure the mentally handicapped but it will certainly improve the quality of their lives.

The progress made in the last 30 years in developing methods of training for the mentally handicapped, even the severely mentally handicapped, should dispel for ever the belief that these people will inevitably be incompetent, and must therefore be over-protected and without opportunity for development.

I would like to thank all the authors for their co-operation in rearranging and modifying their chapters to meet the objectives and aims of what I hope will be a useful and practical text.

Finally, I must thank the publishers, MTP Press Ltd, for their tolerance and patience, my secretary, and other British Institute of Mental Handicap staff who have assisted with the typing of drafts.

G. B. SIMON
Editor

FOREWORD
P. Mittler

This is a book by practitioners for practitioners. Its authors work daily with people who are mentally handicapped and their knowledge and commitment spring from every page.

A practitioners' manual is badly needed because knowledge of good practice is nothing like as widespread as it might be. We need to disseminate good practice by every means at our disposal – not only by books but by films and videorecordings and, above all, by programmes of staff training in the settings in which people work. Staff training is undoubtedly the key to a better service.

This book describes briefly and in simple language what staff actually do in their day-to-day work and it succeeds in conveying a vivid picture of treatment programmes in action. It will undoubtedly be useful to staff working in the service but it should also be read by those outside the service who would like to increase their understanding of recent developments in the field of mental handicap. Since such staff will in future come increasingly into contact with mentally handicapped people, it is obviously important that they should have opportunities to learn about the significant advances that are being made. It is equally important that such opportunities should also be available to policy makers, planners and administrators at national and local level who often determine the resources that will be allocated to mental handicap services.

The book could just as usefully be read by parents and families. Although more parents are now working in partnership with professionals, they do not always receive clear explanations of the range of treatments that are now being used or the reasons why they are thought to be useful. There are still many bridges to be built between parents and professionals and some of the chapters in this book should prove invaluable for this purpose, just as the chapters on the needs of parents contain important material for professionals.

The book also richly illustrates how the treatment of mentally handicapped people demands a multidisciplinary approach. The authors write as skilled practitioners in their own fields but also show a deep awareness and appreciation of the work of their colleagues in other disciplines whose work complements their own. There are still many problems of teamwork to be solved, one of the most basic being that of recruiting scarce professionals into the service and another of ensuring that their skills are available in both health and local authority settings. Here again, the chapters should serve to convey a positive picture of the advances that can be made and stimulate the crossing of professional and administrative boundaries.

There can be no doubt that major advances have been made in the treatment of mentally handicapped people during the last ten years and that further advances in the next decade are possible. There seems to be a much broader base of agreement about what we should be doing and what a good mental handicap service looks like. But it would be dishonest to minimize the difficulties that lie ahead. The chronic shortage of resources which has affected both health and local authority services seems set not only to continue but to become worse. This is all the more frustrating to staff at the very time when they feel that better methods of care and treatment are within their grasp.

It is therefore more important than ever that practitioners present a united front and demonstrate through their work with mentally handicapped people that this long-neglected field deserves a greater share of scarce resources. Too many people in high places still have pessimistic attitudes about the possibilities of achieving results in the field of mental handicap. If we are to make progress in the next ten years, we shall have to convince others as well as ourselves. This book will make an important contribution by showing what can be done.

1

INTRODUCTION: SOME INFORMATION ABOUT MENTAL HANDICAP

G. B. Simon

TERMS

The term 'mental handicap' has generally been used in this book although the following are also in common use:

amentia
mental subnormality
mental deficiency
mental retardation
intellectual retardation

The Mental Health Act of 1959 used the terms 'mental subnormality' and 'severe mental subnormality' described as follows:

Subnormality means a state of arrested or incomplete development of mind (not amounting to 'severe subnormality'), which includes subnormality of intelligence, and is of a nature or degree which requires or is susceptible to medical treatment or other special care or training of the patient.

Severe subnormality means a state of arrested or incomplete development of mind, which includes subnormality of intelligence, and is of such a nature or degree that the patient is incapable of living an independent life or of guarding himself against serious exploitation, or will be so incapable when of an age to do so.

1

The American Association on Mental Deficiency in 1973 referred to it as 'significantly sub-average intellectual functioning existing concurrently with defects in adaptive behaviour and manifested during the developmental period', the upper limit of the latter period being regarded as 18 years.

The criteria used to differentiate the two degrees of subnormality are based in the former on the ability of the individual to care for himself with suitable training, while in severe mental subnormality the individual is regarded as unlikely ever to reach this level of competence.

In most definitions, although 'intelligence' as estimated by standard intelligence tests is mentioned it is not the only facet which influences the ability of an individual to live independently in the community. This is the composite functioning of personality attention, concentration, application, behaviour and intelligence – all of which, or any of which, may be affected in various ways by damage to the brain.

THE FUNCTIONS OF THE BRAIN

Damage to the brain affects certain functions, depending on which part of the brain is affected. Parts of the brain serve specific functions, and arrested or incomplete development of parts which do not include the motor areas, for instance, may leave the person mentally handicapped without physical disability; or damage to motor areas may cause physical defects without affecting the mental functions. Where damage is widespread both mental and physical functions may be affected, and this multiple affliction is seen more frequently in those suffering from severe mental subnormality.

CAUSES OF MENTAL HANDICAP

There is no single disease which causes all mental handicap, and although causes can be identified in about a half to two-thirds of mentally handicapped people, no precise cause has as yet been found in the rest. An awareness of the condition causing mental handicap in an individual is important, as it will influence not only the treatment and management but may also indicate what preventive measures may be taken. These matters will be dealt with in the chapter on causes and prevention.

INCIDENCE OF SEVERE MENTAL HANDICAP

Most surveys in the United Kingdom now suggest that the incidence of severe mental handicap is between three and four per 1000 population with some variation at different ages. About one-third suffer from Down's syndrome (Mongolism).

MENTAL HANDICAP, MENTAL ILLNESS, MENTAL DISORDER

Mental handicap is a state in which the normal intellectual functions of the brain have not fully developed for one reason or another. Alternatively, functions acquired have been lost due to damage or disease before the end of the developmental period; usually the age of 18 years.

Mental illness is a disturbance of the usual mental state of the individual, whatever the actual level might be. In mental illness, therefore, it is the stability and balance of function which is disturbed and disorganized. The quality and extent of this disturbance will depend on the type of mental illness.

The term 'mental disorder' as used in the Mental Health Act 1959 embraces both mental illness and mental handicap. The inclusion of the mentally handicapped in this Act has been under discussion for some time and there are many who feel it should not be included (DHSS, 1976). This will be further discussed in the chapter on the legal aspects of mental handicap.

INCIDENCE OF PSYCHIATRIC DISORDERS

In a survey by Corbett (1979), of 140 severely mentally handicapped children examined, 47% were found to have additional psychiatric problems and of 402 adults examined 46% had psychiatric disorders. It is clear therefore that there is a greater incidence of psychiatric disorder among the mentally handicapped than is the case in the general population. Further details are provided on this in other chapters.

NEEDS OF THE MENTALLY HANDICAPPED

Comprehensive Assessment

All too often in the past this consisted of a half-hour intelligence test, the aim of which was to facilitate an administrative decision on placement. In the chapters of this book dealing with various aspects of mental handicap, authors refer to assessment and describe the methods that are used. Any meaningful comprehensive assessment must include all aspects of the physical and mental state of the individual. In the case of multiply-handicapped children and adults long periods of observation by skilled and experienced staff, coupled with diagnostic teaching and training, will frequently be necessary if the programmes that should follow are to be of any real benefit.

Programmes of Treatment and Management

Although it is essential to find a cause, if possible, and assess the level of ability of the mentally handicapped person it is equally important, after the areas of deficit have been identified, to devise a programme enabling the individual to make whatever improvement is possible. Diagnosis on its own is necessary for the reasons already mentioned, but it will not help the handicapped individual himself unless it is followed by the appropriate programme of treatment; this being reviewed and revised at regular intervals.

Most of the essential services required by the young handicapped child, including those who are mentally handicapped, should be available through the paediatric services at District General Hospitals. If and when these services are not able to deal with the problems of individual mentally handicapped children, and this is frequently because of the associated psychiatric and behaviour problems, the National Development Group and Development Team suggest that referral should be made to a Specialised Community Team. These teams consist of the part-time or full-time services of medical, psychological, social and nursing specialists with access to the services of others, and are now being established for areas with populations of 60 000–80 000. The functions, role and composition of these teams are described in detail in reports by the Developmental Team for the Mentally

4

Handicapped (1976/7 and 1978/9) and are referred to repeatedly elsewhere in this book.

References

Corbett, J. A. (1979). *Psychiatric Illness and Mental Handicap*. (London: Gaskell Press)

DHSS (Department of Health & Social Security) (1976). *A Review of the Mental Health Act*. (London: HMSO)

Developmental Team for the Mentally Handicapped. Reports 1976/7 and 1978/9. (London: HMSO)

2

CAUSES AND PREVENTION

J. Jancar and G. B. Simon

CAUSES

The prevalence of severe mental handicap has been between 3 and 5 per 1000 with only minor variations for the past 30 years and these differences are probably the result of differences in criteria, ascertainment and notification. In about two-thirds of those suffering from severe mental handicap some indication of the cause can be established.

It is not intended here to provide exhaustive lists of conditions associated with mental handicap but to indicate to the reader in general terms when and how mental handicap comes about and provide some understanding of preventive programmes. Further information on the causes of mental handicap can be obtained from the more detailed texts in the reading list at the end of this chapter.

Before Birth

The characteristics of individuals are inherited from their parents through the germ cells (male sperm and female egg) which come together at conception. Disorders which result from deficiencies and abnormalities of this genetic material are, therefore, establish-ed at this time and although some may be evident in pregnancy, others may not show until birth or after. One of the best known of the chromosomal abnormalities is Down's syndrome which ac-counts for about one-third of severe mental handicap.

Other inherited conditions include a number of biochemical disorders accounting for about 4–5%. These affect the breakdown and use of proteins, carbohydrates and fats and are due to a lack of one or more of the essential enzymes required for these substances, which are essential for normal development to be utilized. Mental handicap also results from infections in pregnancy, for although the uterus offers good protection, some organisms can pass through it to the developing child and of these, although rubella is probably the best known, there are other virus diseases which are, in fact, more frequent. Congenital syphilis decreased in pregnancy with the advent of antibiotics. However, recently the incidence appears to be on an increase.

Spina bifida is a condition which gives rise to a number of defects of the central nervous system (the brain and spinal cord) present before birth. Drugs such as thalidomide and other sub-stances such as lead, if present in significant quantity in the mother's circulation may also affect the child. Many conditions in the mother such as anaemia, high blood pressure, some kidney and liver diseases and diabetes may also affect the child. Bleeding in pregnancy may, if it is massive and repeated, also reduce the blood supply to the child. Most of these diseases affect the developing child in the womb by reducing the oxygen-carrying capacity of the blood and, therefore, deprive the developing baby of essential oxygen.

Disorders of mother's endocrine glands such as the pituitary, thyroid or adrenal glands can have a secondary effect on the child by depriving it of an essential for development or through a lack of the stimulation which is essential for the baby's own glandular development.

Alcohol has now been shown to affect the unborn child when drunk to excess by the pregnant woman, causing severe mental retardation associated with a number of congenital physical ab-normalities.

Similarly excessive smoking during pregnancy can impair normal physical and mental development of the fetus.

Radiation due to X-ray or from the other sources, particularly from seven to fifteen weeks of pregnancy can cause mental and physical handicap.

At Birth and Just After

Prematurity refers to the baby born before its time when its organs are immature and unable to sustain or meet its needs and under these circumstances without very specialized services to overcome this may also result in severe mental handicap. The same situation applies in multiple pregnancies when more than one baby is in the womb and when they may be small and underweight. At birth there is also the possibility of injury to the brain, from a variety of causes both through direct mechanical damage and also through factors in the environment.

Haemolytic disease or destruction of the baby's blood resulting in severe jaundice can bring about physical handicap such as cerebral palsy and mental handicap.

Lack of thyroid in the baby is another condition which may become evident very early in life and if not remedied can give rise to maldevelopment and mental handicap.

Encephalitis and meningitis which are infections of the brain itself and its coverings may occur when the brain can be damaged. In the past 10 years the discovery and increasing availability of antibiotics has diminished this. For instance, tuberculous meningitis, a potent cause of brain damage and relatively common in children 40 years ago, is now rare as a result of a decrease in tuberculosis itself.

Defects of the heart which diminish its efficiency and reduce the oxygen supply to the brain also bring about its maldevelopment.

Post-natal Period

This period usually extends to the end of the second year and during this time, infections continue to be a possibility and can result in meningitis and encephalitis. Many of these are also now less of a problem because of the availability of antibiotics.

Some infections, previously almost eliminated through vaccination and inoculation are now reappearing due to lack of adherence to programmes of prevention, frequently the result of the fears of parents that these measures may in themselves cause the damage they are intended to eliminate.

There are conditions which are known to be associated with mental handicap, for example, tuberous sclerosis or epiloia in which severe epilepsy occurs accompanied by maldevelopment and damage to the brain. The causes of some of these conditions are not at present known with certainty although it has been established that they cause arrested or incomplete development of the brain.

Accidental and non-accidental injuries which cause fractures of the skull, haemorrhage and brain damage are also important in the cause of mental and multiple handicap.

Severe gastroenteritis which causes dehydration during early childhood if not treated may result in brain damage sufficient to cause mental handicap which might be accompanied by spasticity and epilepsy.

PREVENTION

It has been estimated that over a third of the handicap identified in the first year of life originated in the period of early pregnancy. Genetic conditions, for instance, originate at this period as do the effects of certain drugs. Infections such as rubella, which is a mild condition in itself and frequently passes unnoticed can, if it occurs in the first 3 months of pregnancy, in a mother who has no immunity to it, be transmitted to the developing fetus and can cause a number of severe multiple congenital abnormalities including severe mental handicap.

The following are among the most widely practised and effective preventive measures:

1. Programmes of inoculation and vaccination in children and adults so that immunity is acquired to the organisms which are responsible for the infections that cause encephalitis and meningitis. For instance, in the case of rubella, every woman should be tested at least 3 months before an intending pregnancy for immunity and if required should be vaccinated.

In the case of those who lack immunity but are already pregnant, they should be vaccinated after delivery.

Where a woman is found to be Rhesus negative, it is now possible to immunize her against the development of antibodies during her first pregnancy and to prevent damage to later children.

2. Publicity has been given in recent years both in the medical and lay press to possible effects on the developing child of certain drugs and other substances so that many of these causes should now be avoided if adequate programmes of education and antenatal care are carried out.

3. Improved surveillance in pregnancy also ensures that monitoring of the baby's development in the womb takes place and in the case of some metabolic diseases will enable the relevant tests to be carried out so that conditions such as diabetes and other errors in metabolism can be discovered and controlled.

4. As a shortage of oxygen and low birth weight in babies are an important cause of mental handicap, improved antenatal and perinatal care associated with the availability of the expertise to anticipate these problems and remedy them without delay is an obvious measure in prevention. The delivery of some 96% of babies in hospital or nursing homes (Department of Health and Social Security, 1977) where paediatric services are available with facilities for immediate intervention if necessary, should eliminate some of the complications which lead to brain damage.

5. A preventive step now available for at least some who may be born with Down's syndrome, many biochemical abnormalities and spina bifida, is the possibility of diagnosis during pregnancy through examination of the amniotic fluid which surrounds the baby in the womb. It is known that about 30% of children with Down's syndrome are born to mothers between 35 and 40 years of age. Although the majority (about 70%) of these children are born to younger mothers without a previous history, nevertheless, if mothers over the age of 35 are offered these facilities for diagnosis in pregnancy, some of these births could be avoided.

6. All prospective parents with a family history or evidence of a genetically transmitted abnormality should have access to

11

genetic counselling. This should also apply to anyone who wishes to get genetic advice.

7. Social and living standards and efficient diet are general aspects of life, the effects of which are difficult to assess but which may affect the development of the child.

IMPLICATIONS OF PREVENTIVE PROGRAMMES

Programmes of prevention, however simple they may appear, have administrative, ethical, moral, social and economic implications which will affect their outcome. The screening of a woman in pregnancy and discovery of a disabling condition in the unborn child is not in itself preventive of handicap and must be followed by the next logical step, which may be a therapeutic abortion, or the instigation of treatment during pregnancy if this is possible or soon after birth if the condition is treatable.

The adoption of programmes of prevention by most Governments will depend on establishing clearly that it is cost-effective and this will depend on a number of factors, two of which are most important, i.e. the efficiency with which it is operated and its acceptance by the people who must use it if it is to be successful.

In theory, if a programme were instituted to study every pregnancy where the mother is over 35 years of age it could prove effective in avoiding 30% of Down's syndrome babies being born. This, however, depends on every vulnerable person agreeing to the investigation and subsequently consenting to a therapeutic abortion if the diagnosis is confirmed. Every step is fraught with ifs and buts. Will *all* mothers in this group be known and included? Will *all* agree to investigation? Would those with positive findings consent to a therapeutic abortion? Positive answers to these questions cannot be ensured very easily in a democratic society, although ultimately the cost-effectiveness of the programme will depend on them.

One measure which has been financed and given much publicity since 1970 is the use of rubella vaccine on school girls at 11 to 13 years of age to ensure that all women have acquired immunity before pregnancy. The acceptance or the 'take-up rate' of this offer, however, varies from 40% to 90% in different parts of the

United Kingdom. In addition the precautions and steps necessary for effective administration of the vaccine to ensure success, such as the maintenance of supplies at the correct temperature or non-exposure to light are still not clearly understood by some of the staff using it even after 4 years of wide practice.

It is clear, therefore, that however successful any programme could be in theory, its ultimate success depends on a number of other factors and variables, not least of which is a very considerable human element.

In spite of the difficulties that are inherent in almost every programme of prevention, not least of which is the human element involved, they must be encouraged and use made of the advances in antenatal diagnosis and immunological techniques that are becoming increasingly available. This does not mean that every measure suggested should be accepted without thorough evaluation but having taken every step possible to ensure its effectiveness and safety. It is essential that the publicity exercise and accompanying instruction should be convincing and wholehearted if it is to be accepted and serve its ultimate purpose which is the prevention of handicap and disability.

Further Reading

Prevention and Health (1977). Command Paper 7047 (London: HMSO)

Reducing the Risk (1977). (London: HMSO)

Craft, M. (1979). *Tredgold's Mental Retardation*, 12th Edn. (London: Baillière Tindall)

Symposium on the cost of preventing major mental handicap; Methods and costs of prevention. Symposium 59 CIBA Foundation (1977) (Amsterdam: Elsevier)

Eastham, R.D. and Jancar, J. (1968). *Clinical Pathology in Mental Retardation*. (Bristol: John Wright & Sons)

3

GENETICS AND MENTAL HANDICAP

V. A. Cowie

The implications of genetics in mental handicap are so far-reaching that within the space of a single chapter it is impossible to achieve more than an outline of the underlying principles of genetic causation and a review of their practical application. Aspects which merit particular attention have been selected; these include the need for accurate diagnosis, the interpretation to parents of degree of genetic risk, problems and hazards in genetic counselling and the vital matter of the initial disclosure to parents of the diagnosis of a genetic condition. Prenatal diagnosis of genetic conditions is of special significance in connection with mental handicap, and its positive aspects, besides its value as a tool in preventive medicine, are discussed.

BASIC GENETIC PRINCIPLES

In considering the contribution of genetics to the causation of mental handicap, it is useful to have in mind three important categories of genetic transmission; these are:

polygenic inheritance;
genetic transmission by means of rare single genes of major effect;

15

the effect of numerical or morphological changes in the chromosomes.

The first two modes of inheritance are mainly deduced from the pattern in the family pedigree created by the distribution of affected members in the family tree. The genes themselves cannot be seen, and are believed to be the arrangement of chemical components of the DNA molecule at specific loci on the chromosomes. On the other hand, in the third category, comparatively gross changes have taken place involving whole chromosomes or parts of chromosomes; these are detectable under the microscope using cytogenetic techniques.

It is important to understand basic genetic principles because upon them rests the advice that can be given in genetic counselling, particularly as regards the risk of recurrence of a condition in subsequent offspring.

Polygenic Inheritance

Polygenic inheritance is responsible to a large extent for the variation in the distribution of human intelligence; therefore it is responsible for that proportion of mental handicap which can be regarded as the lower end of the normal range of distribution of intelligence in the general population. Like other biological variables such as stature, intelligence shows continuous variation through any random population. If an individual in a sufficiently large population were to be measured for characteristics such as stature or intelligence, the difference between the measurement of one individual and the next on a graded scale is so very small that when the measurements of the whole group are plotted, a steady, smooth gradation is seen without any sharp fluctuations. Furthermore, a curve is obtained which is approximately symmetrical about a peak at the mean, dropping off either side to produce the well-known bell shape of the Gaussian curve of normal distribution, which has an exact mathematical formula. The continuous variation seen in such 'normal distribution' is due to the additive effect of many factors, each of small effect. These factors are both environmental and genetic; the genetic elements here are called polygenes: for this reason the genetic component is known as polygenic inheritance. However, because of the interaction of environmental factors, which are very important in the determination of normal distribution, the term multifactorial is sometimes preferred to polygenic in connection with the elements of causation.

Regarding intelligence as a biological variable showing continuous variation, it covers an unbroken range from superior levels and genius at one extreme to backwardness and subnormality of increasing severity at the other. In this way mental subnormality may arise as an extreme expression of a biological variable of multifactorial or polygenic causation. However, this accounts for mental handicap only in a proportion of cases; the curve of normal distribution for intelligence is not absolutely symmetrical, but shows an asymmetry at the extreme lower end of the scale, being affected by a number of individuals in excess of that expected by normal distribution alone. The severe mental subnormality in the case of these individuals is due to major single causative factors, either genetic or environmental, rather than having multifactorial causation. The major single genetic factors are the rare single genes of major effect, and chromosome aberrations.

· Rare Single Genes of Major Effect

Single genes of major damaging effect associated with mental handicap are fortunately very rare. Their presence can be inferred by the pattern of manifestation of a specific condition in a family, but a number of affected individuals may not have inherited the gene from one or both parents: in their case the gene will have arisen *de novo* as a fresh mutation. Once the gene has come into being in this way it will be transmissible to the descendants of its possessor, following the pattern characteristic for that particular gene.

The modes of inheritance of these rare single genes are often referred to as Mendelian, having been observed and described by Mendel over 100 years ago. They are of two kinds: dominant and recessive, and most are autosomal dominant or autosomal recessive. This means that they are carried on a chromosome which is not a sex chromosome; i.e. an autosome. Some genes,

17

however, are carried on an X chromosome in the sex chromosome pair on the part of that chromosome that is not matched by the Y chromosome; these are known as sex-linked.

A dominant trait is one which shows itself when the gene is present in heterozygous form. The chromosomes are paired; therefore the genes upon them are paired. When one gene only of the pair is abnormal, through mutation in the individual bearing it or in an ancestor from whom it has been transmitted, then the gene is said to be present in heterozygous form and its possessor is a heterozygote. Dominance is recognized in families by continued transmission from parent to child. The theoretical genetic risk of the gene being passed to a child is of the order of 50%. Dominant genes have, in general, a high mutation rate; often a dominant condition is seen having arisen *de novo* in an individual neither of whose parents or, indeed, any antecedents, have shown any signs of the condition. Dominant conditions are often extremely variable in their manifestation in one family; some members may be severely affected, others only mildly, and the number and pattern of clinical signs may vary from one relative to another. Tuberous sclerosis and acrocephaly are examples of conditions associated with mental handicap which are caused by autosomal dominant genes.

Autosomal recessive genes, in contradistinction, are characterized by the necessity for them to be present in homozygous form before the condition becomes manifest to its fullest extent. The homozygote, who possesses such a pair of abnormal genes, will have inherited one gene of the pair from each parent. The parents are possessors of the gene in single dose; heterozygotes. They, and other carriers of the gene in single dose, usually show no apparent abnormality, but certain biochemical and cytological tests are available for detecting the carrier state in some recessive conditions. The inborn errors of metabolism, which constitute a large group of rare conditions such as phenylketonuria, galactosaemia and maple syrup urine disease, are nearly all autosomal recessive conditions. The theoretical risk for a pair of parents who are heterozygous for an autosomal recessive condition, and who probably have shown themselves to be so by already producing an affected child, stands at approximately 25% (or one in four) for producing a child similarly affected in subsequent pregnancies.

Sex-linked genes are carried on the X chromosome and if recessive, the conditions associated with them are manifested only in the male but are transmitted by apparently unaffected female carriers. Such a female carrier stands at a theoretical risk of having 50% of her sons affected, while the remaining 50% may be expected to be normal. Sex-linked conditions are very much rarer than conditions due to autosomal dominant or recessive genes. Examples of sex-linked conditions associated with mental handicap are Hunter's syndrome (a form of gargoylism: mucopolysaccharidosis type II), and the Lesch–Nyhan syndrome (hyperuricacidaemia).

Chromosome Abnormalities

Mongolism, or Down's syndrome, was the first abnormal human condition recognized to have an association with a chromosome anomaly demonstrable by microscopic techniques. About twenty years ago, Lejeune and his team in Paris showed this condition to be associated with an abnormal chromosome pattern, or karyotype, in which an extra chromosome was present. In most cases the extra chromosome is lying free, and appears (when the photographed chromosomes are arranged according to convention) to be additional to one of the pairs of the smallest autosomal chromosomes in the human cell complement, traditionally designated chromosome 21. This state is described as trisomic. In a small proportion (probably somewhat less than 3%) of patients with Down's syndrome, the extra chromosome is fused with another, in the so-called translocated state. This may arise as a fresh mutation, a kind of genetic accident, in which case the parents may be expected to have normal karyotypes. Not infrequently, however, one of the parents of a patient with the translocation type of Down's syndrome is found to possess the translocated chromosome in a balanced form, and in the family of such an individual, relatives may be found also to be balanced carriers. Balanced carriers of a translocation of this kind stand a calculable genetic risk of producing an affected child. It is therefore necessary to identify them and give them the opportunity for genetic counselling. The starting point of this exercise is the ascertainment of whether or not the patient with Down's syndrome has a chromosomal translocation or whether his condition is due to the more common trisomy. It is therefore of very practical purpose, and indeed a clinical obligation, to identify the karyotype of a patient with Down's syndrome. Down's syndrome is much more common than the very rare single-gene defects, and is, indeed, the commonest syndrome which is associated with mental handicap and which arises in conjunction with an abnormality of an autosomal chromosome. Its rate of occurrence has been estimated at about one in every 666 live births (Carter and MacCarthy, 1951).

An association with specific chromosome defects has been discovered in many other conditions of mental handicap. Trisomy and chromosomal translocation have already been referred to; in these there is an excess of chromosomal material. In some chromosome defects there may be a deletion of chromosomal material, in which a part of a chromosome may be seen to be missing. An example of a condition associated with a chromosomal deletion is the cri-du-chat (cat's cry) syndrome, in which a small part of chromosome no. 5 is missing.

Chromosome abnormalities involving autosomal chromosomes are, in general, associated with severe mental handicap and widespread physical changes. On the other hand, sex chromosome abnormalities are associated on the whole with mental deficit of lesser degree, although the level of mental functioning may vary considerably from one individual to another. The physical changes are also less marked, on the whole, than those associated with autosomal chromosome abnormalities, but the brunt of anatomical changes falls generally on the gonads and genital tract. Various psychiatric changes have been described in association with sex chromosome abnormalities in addition to impairment in cognitive functioning; these in the main appear to affect character and personality when they occur.

THE DISCLOSURE OF DIAGNOSIS OF A GENETIC CONDITION

In genetic conditions associated with mental handicap, especially if the condition is recognizable at birth, as in the case of Down's syndrome, the first task in genetic counselling usually is to break the news to the parents. The way in which this task is undertaken is of the utmost importance; if handled with ineptitude the consequences may be disastrous. Faulty timing, clumsy handling and insensitivity to the feelings of the parents may profoundly affect the attitude of those parents to their mentally handicapped child.

In the past there has been much difference of opinion as to the optimum time for disclosure. A great many doctors favoured withholding this information, presumably in the hope that the truth would gradually dawn on the parents and that this would be preferable to the sudden shock of an early revelation.

Although kindly meant, such procrastination has often brought much more distress to parents than straightforward early disclosure. The truth in such cases seldom dawns slowly. More often, it is brought to the parents' notice suddenly in an unfortunate way and without the supporting information that is so necessary. For example, unsuspecting mothers have been told for the first time by neighbours or even by casual bystanders in the street that their child is a mongol. Even without this experience, the spontaneous realization that a child is mentally handicapped can be a severe shock. Up to that time they will have believed their child to be normal; they will have created an illusory picture of its future life and expectations, and the sudden dashing of these hopes, built up over a period of time, can be catastrophic.

The practice of delaying the disclosure is less in evidence today. This may be partly due to a greater public awareness of the nature of mental handicap and its implications. Parents are less reticent in asking questions of their doctors. Public awareness of clinical and genetic topics has been increased by television programmes and other sources, and it is to be hoped that these media will be used to advantage to bring further enlightenment. Already this good influence is being felt, and with the demand by parents for more precise information comes the demand to be told early and truthfully if a child is mentally subnormal.

A number of studies have been made bearing out the desirability of early disclosure of the condition with parents of a mongol baby. In a study by the writer of this chapter (Cowie, 1966) one or both parents, out of 51 pairs to whom a child with Down's syndrome had been born, were asked at what stage they felt it was best for the first information about the child's condition to be given. No fewer than 41 pairs of parents from the whole group of 51 pairs said 'at birth' or 'at once' or 'as soon as the doctors are sure of the diagnosis'. These findings are in accordance with those of Drillien and Wilkinson (1964) who investigated a series of 70 mothers of babies with Down's syndrome. They found that the mothers who spoke most appreciatively were those who were warned or told soon after birth, and were thereafter given the opportunity for regular support and advice.

When a child dies in infancy the most common reaction of average young parents is to consider having another baby as soon as possible. If the dead child had a condition associated with mental handicap, a full explanation of the condition and genetic counselling are urgent matters.

CAUTION IN THE INTERPRETATION OF SIGNS AND THE APPLICATION OF GENERAL GENETIC PRINCIPLES

Carter (1971) says that when the geneticist makes mistakes in counselling, it is most often from errors in diagnosis. He goes on to point out that when the clinician makes mistakes it is because he does not know a condition may be inherited in more than one way, or that empirical risk figures are available when the genetics of the condition are complex. The ideal counsellor is someone with a sound knowledge both of genetics and of the particular field of medicine.

Accuracy of diagnosis is an essential prerequisite for genetic counselling. No pains should be spared in examination of the patient (if alive and available). A careful family history should be taken. Detailed clinical information about affected relatives should be obtained, and if possible these relatives should be seen and examined. Special investigations of affected family members may be called for, such as amino-acid screening for inborn errors of metabolism, or chromosome investigations. It is advisable to obtain all relevant data in order to arrive at a precise diagnosis before embarking upon actual counselling.

As regards many patients for whose mental handicap no diagnosis can be reached and no clue can be found to the aetiology, Berg and Kirman (1959) found that approximately 60% of patients in a sample from a hospital for the severely mentally subnormal remained completely unclassified. In such cases, genetic counselling rests on empirical risk figures. A figure of approximately 3% risk for recurrence in the relatives of such unclassified patients was reached by analysis of systematically collated family data from this hospital population.

DEGREE OF RISK AND ATTITUDE OF PARENTS

The empirical risk figure of about 3% just quoted for the recurrence of abnormality in the sibs of unclassified patients is a very low risk, only three times the random risk for the general population. High-risk situations arise in connection with a small proportion of chromosome anomalies, and with conditions associated with a single gene of major effect (dominant, recessive, autosomal and sex-linked conditions). The small proportion of chromosome anomalies carrying a high risk are mainly structural anomalies, such as translocations, which may be carried in a balanced state in the cells of a clinically normal parent. When this is found, chromosome investigations of relatives of such a parent may be called for, so that other carriers in the family can be alerted to the genetic risk. The risk for different kinds of anomaly of this sort appears to be variable, but the order of risk can be exemplified by the translocation in Down's syndrome in which the greater part of one chromosome is fused with that of another. Sometimes this translocation arises as a fresh mutation in a patient and the chromosome patterns of the parents then appear to be normal. However, if the mother has the translocation in balanced form, the risk of her having an affected child may be about one in five; but when the father has it, probably the risk is less than one in twenty. These theoretical risk figures are dependent upon which chromosomes are involved in the translocation; this can be ascertained by cytogenetic analysis.

Moderate-risk situations arise in connection with conditions with a complex hereditary predisposition that can be seen by familial recurrence in large-scale family studies. On the basis of such studies, statistical risk figures can be estimated. There may be some variation of risk according to geographical or racial distribution. For example on the basis of family studies the recurrence risk in South Wales of a neural tube malformation, spina bifida or anencephaly but not primary hydrocephalus, has been calculated as about one in sixteen, but in south east England it is probably somewhat less; probably one in twenty-five (Carter, 1971). The risk increases for mothers who have had two children with such malformations, and is probably of the order of one in eight (Carter and Roberts, 1967).

A primary objective in genetic counselling is to give parents information about the degree of genetic risk. This is often further clarified if the mode of inheritance can be explained in everyday terms to the parents. McBean (1971), with reference to phenylketonuria, says that this is meaningless to people of simple intelligence and that few can be expected to understand the recessive mode of inheritance if they have already had two or more affected children, or know of other families where this exists. My own experience is at variance with this. By explaining the genetic risk in very simple terms such as betting odds that apply to each birth as a single independent event as opposed to the expected proportions in families of affected children, very few parents fail to grasp what is meant. Often by drawing simple diagrams one can explain the elements of gene transmission or even more complicated genetical matters such as chromosomal translocation. Parents are usually grateful not only for this information but for any pains taken to enlighten them about a subject which concerns them vitally but which is usually regarded as too abstruse and esoteric for general explanation.

Once the parents have been given an assessment of genetic risk, it is entirely up to them to make decisions; for example, regarding having further children. This is a personal matter and the genetic counsellor can only give guidelines to help them to make their own decision. Many factors can influence their course of action. Important amongst these are social factors such as the presence of a handicapped child already in the family, creating many demands or psychological factors such as the fear of having another affected child, even if the risk is only minimally increased.

PRENATAL DIAGNOSIS BY AMNIOCENTESIS: AN EXTENSION OF GENETIC COUNSELLING

The means of detection of various genetically determined conditions in the fetus has brought a new dimension to genetic counselling in mental handicap. It is possible to detect chromosome anomalies in fetal cells extracted from amniotic fluid obtained by amniotic puncture (amniocentesis).

Amniocentesis is carried out by tapping the fluid with a special needle through the abdominal wall. The needle must pierce through the skin and underlying tissues and musculature, through the wall of the uterus and amniotic sac; therefore scrupulous care must be taken as regards aseptic precautions. Prior to the puncture the lie of the fetus and position of the placenta and other structures should be determined by sonography to avoid puncturing a structure such as a large vessel; ensuing haemorrhage could be a hazard. Another risk of amniocentesis is the precipitation of premature labour, with loss of the fetus. The overall risk of the procedure, however, is small in skilled hands and in proper conditions and, as will be indicated, various surveys have showed the overall risk to the pregnancy in amniocentesis to be small. The optimum time for amniocentesis is around the fourteenth to sixteenth week of pregnancy. By this time the uterus is sufficiently high above the rim of the pelvis for a transabdominal puncture to be made, and early enough for a repeat puncture should this be necessary for technical reasons.

` This procedure is especially useful in situations such as those involving chromosome translocations, when one of the parents may be a balanced carrier. Such parents, who otherwise might prefer to avoid having further children, may now go ahead, knowing that if the fetus is found to be affected, termination of the pregnancy is available. In any situation, indeed, in which it is considered that the pregnant mother may stand at particular risk for producing a child with a chromosome abnormality, it is advisable for prenatal diagnosis by amniocentesis to be considered. As regards chromosome abnormalities, it is well known that mothers becoming pregnant late in the reproductive period are at special risk for producing an affected child. The late maternal age factor is particularly well known in connection with Down's syndrome. In a number of centres, including our own, amniocentesis is offered to women becoming pregnant at the age of 40 or over. In some, the age threshold is lower at 35 years or over. The fixing of an age threshold is determined largely by the resources available to meet the work-load.

It is possible to diagnose certain inborn errors of metabolism by measuring specific enzyme activity of the fetal cells. So far, this has been successful in a limited number of conditions, including Tay Sachs disease (infantile amaurotic idiocy), and the Lesch–Nyhan syndrome (hyperuricacidaemia). The techniques involved call for a high degree of expertise and are available only in certain centres. They are being evolved by systematic research. This underlines the need for the support and extension of medical research upon whose results the very practical aid to many families depends.

The withdrawal of amniotic fluid is not without some risk. The risks, however, are small, and the total risk has been estimated at less than 1% (Gerbie et al., 1971; Kalbac and Newman, 1974). A slightly higher figure of 3.3% of fetal death through abortion on amniocentesis has been the experience of Polani and his team in the Paediatric Research Unit at Guy's Hospital (Polani, 1977, Personal communication). Indeed very extensive studies (Canadian Research Council, 1977; Editorial, British Medical Journal, 1977) show no significant difference in fetal loss among pregnant women undergoing amniocentesis as compared with matched controls. Therefore the risk in experienced hands is small, but it should be discussed with the pregnant mother and her husband if amniocentesis is being considered.

If amniocentesis is to be considered, it is important not to leave it too late. This is brought home in the study by Duncan (1978). In her study a first appearance at the hospital by an estimated 20 weeks gestation was taken as the absolute limit for initiating the procedure, though around 16 weeks was the preferred time. The most striking feature in this study was that about half the women booked too late for the procedure to be considered. The main factors appeared to be failure in communication and late booking.

The prenatal diagnosis of neural tube defects (open spina bifida and anencephaly) is now possible by estimation of the alphafetoprotein (AFP) in the amniotic fluid. This is significantly raised in the presence of such abnormalities in the fetus. Progress is being made in the use of maternal serum levels of AFP for preliminary screening, with a view to undertaking amniocentesis in the case of those mothers in whom the maternal serum AFP is significantly high. This is an important development in preventive medicine and for mental handicap which is concomitant with severe neural tube defects.

THE CO-ORDINATION OF GENETIC SERVICES

Up to now, genetic counselling services in the United Kingdom have been developed mainly through the efforts of individuals with a special interest in medical genetics. Consequently these services have grown up in a haphazard way, and do not give adequate national coverage (Cowie, 1977). It is also clear that the medical and allied professions are very poorly equipped on the whole for the front-line management of genetic problems. This became clear in a study involving the parents of children with severe neural tube defects (Cowie *et al.*, 1975, unpublished data). Many of these parents complained of misleading information they had been given, by general practitioners and hospital doctors, about the genetic implications of their child's condition; in a number of instances it appeared that these doctors did not even know where, or to whom, to refer them for genetic advice.

A prerequisite in providing better services is properly organized teaching. Multidisciplinary teaching is to be recommended. It would be especially helpful to have combined courses for medical undergraduates and postgraduates, nurses, social workers, midwives and health visitors. In practice, the co-ordinated work of a team, of which the general practitioner is often the leading figure, together with the social workers and other visiting personnel, is essential in the front-line management and subsequent necessary family support in the home following the birth of a child with a recognizable genetic defect (Emery, 1975). This is an important and often neglected aspect of community medicine. For co-ordinated work of this kind, joint training of the various members of the team, in order to meet these needs, should be a priority in their training curricula. A university-based training service is to be recommended as an ideal for a number of reasons; not least to provide a nexus for such training. A university department could provide special curricula for different categories of workers destined to become members of counselling teams. Multidisciplinary seminars would be especially valuable, and would establish from the beginning a habit and regimen of communication which at present is often so sadly lacking.

At a time when there is rapidly growing public demand parallel with important advances in genetic techniques and expertise, it is appropriate that methods should be considered for putting to the best use the resources at our disposal. This is of prime importance in our efforts to take effective measures in the prevention of mental handicap.

References

Berg, J. and Kirman, B. H. (1959). Some aetiological problems in mental deficiency. *Br. Med. J.*, **2**, 848

Canadian Research Council (1977). *Diagnosis of Genetic Disease by Amniocentesis during the Second Trimester of Pregnancy*. Report No. 5. (Ottawa: Ministry of Supplies and Services)

Carter, C. O. (1971). Genetic counselling. In Berg, J. M. (ed.) *Genetic Counselling in Relation to Mental Retardation*. Symposium No. 2. Institute for Research into Mental Retardation. (Oxford: Pergamon Press)

Carter, C. O. and Roberts, J. A. F. (1967). The risk of recurrence after two children with central nervous system malformations. *Lancet*, **1**, 306

Carter, C. O. and MacCarthy, D. (1951). Incidence of mongolism and its diagnosis in the newborn. *Br. J. Soc. Med.*, **5**, 83

Cowie, V. A. (1966). Genetic Counselling. *Proc. Roy. Soc. Med.*, **59**, 149

Cowie, V. A. (1977). Genetic counselling clinics. In Raine, D. N. (ed.) *Medico-Social Management of Inherited Metabolic Disease*. A monograph derived from the Thirteenth Symposium of the Society for the Study of Inborn Errors of Metabolism, pp. 103–117. (Lancaster: MTP)

Cowie, V. A., Eckstein, H. and Colliss, V. (1975). Unpublished data

Drillien, C. M. and Wilkinson, E. M. (1964). Mongolism: when should parents be told? *Br. Med. J.*, **2**, 1306

Duncan, S. L. B. (1978). Problems of pre-natal screening programme for Down's syndrome in older women. *J. Biosoc. Sci.*, **10**, 141

Editorial, *British Medical Journal* (1977). Diagnostic amniocentesis in early pregnancy. *Br. Med. J.*, **1**, 1430

Emery, A. E. H. (1975). Genetic counselling. *Br. Med. J.*, **ii**, 219

Gerbie, A. B., Nadler, H. L. and Gerbie, M. M. (1971). Amniocentesis in genetic counselling. Safety and reliability in early pregnancy. *Am. J. Obstet. Gynecol.*, **109**, 765

Kalbac, R. W. and Newman, R. L. (1974). Amniotic fluid analysis in complicated pregnancies. *Obstet. Gynecol.*, **44**, 814

McBean, S. (1971). The problems of parents of children with phenylketonuria. In Bichel, H., Hudson, F. P. and Woolf, L. I. (eds.) *Phenylketonuria and Some Other Inborn Errors of Amino-Acid Metabolism*, pp. 280–2. (Stuttgart: Thième)

Polani, P. E. (1977). (Personal communication)

4

MEDICAL TREATMENT OF BEHAVIOUR PROBLEMS IN PEOPLE WITH MENTAL HANDICAP

J. A. Corbett

INTRODUCTION

When the whole population of people with mental retardation in a community is looked at, rather than selected groups receiving particular services, behaviour problems present as the commonest secondary handicap causing difficulty in providing education, training and care. Parents with children at home will see problems different from those seen by staff working in schools, training centres and residential homes or hospitals, and it is not surprising that attitudes to, and experience of, medical treatment vary widely and often give rise to controversy.

The term behaviour disorder is preferable to emotional or psychiatric problem, as it implies a careful description and analysis of the possible causes of the problem.

In the absence of a precise account of the subjective experience, the presence of emotional disorder may only be deduced with difficulty, while the presence of a psychiatric illness implies that a particular constellation of behavioural symptoms or other features are present, and that the problem is amenable to a particular form of treatment. This is a situation which is relatively uncommon in the mentally retarded. It is understandable that a common reaction, when parents begin to realize that their child is handicapped, is to hope for a medical cure. Many attempts have been made to find a simple solution but with a few notable exceptions, such as the use of thyroid hormone to treat cretinism and the dietary treatment of some inborn errors of metabolism such as phenyl-ketonuria, these have not stood up to careful scrutiny (Lipton *et al.*, 1977). Thus treatment with large doses of vitamins, the so-called 'mega-vitamin treatment', extracts of fetal cells (sickle cell therapy) and amino acids such as 5-hydroxytryptophan to improve muscle tone in children with Down's syndrome, are a few among many treatments which have been advocated; initially with enthusiasm. Only after a lapse of time have the effects been systematically evaluated (by comparing the effects of the treatment in a homogeneous group of patients with a carefully matched group not receiving the treatment) and found to be ineffective. Ethical and practical difficulties in carrying out such controlled trials in people with mental handicap have led to a situation where experience with treatments given to ameliorate symptoms, rather than improve learning capacity, has largely been drawn from experience in treating mental illness and behavioural disorders in people of normal intelligence. Knowledge of the effects of drugs in the mentally handicapped is still relatively limited.

Limited facilities, understaffing and lack of alternatives have forced professional staff to look for medical treatments as an alternative to other forms of care. This has led to the taking of polarized views: either that medication is always bad and should be avoided at all costs; or at the other extreme that it should and must be tried for all troublesome behaviour. This leads to the situation that some retarded people who could function better with medication do not receive it, while others who need different types of help may be inappropriately medicated in an attempt to control difficult behaviour.

The difficulty of evaluating medical treatment for behavioural disorders in mental retardation is understandable when we come to look at the multiplicity of factors involved in causing these problems and in accounting for the increased rate of behaviour disorders in people with severe mental handicap. These relationships have been discussed in detail by Rutter (1971) and Corbett (1977) but a brief account will be given here before considering the treatments available.

CAUSES OF BEHAVIOUR DISORDERS

Although behaviour problems are not uncommonly associated with mental retardation, and emotional disturbance can impair intellectual functioning, it is rarely if ever a cause of severe mental retardation on its own. Delayed or impaired cognitive development is generally evident before the onset of behaviour disturbance, and virtually all severely retarded people have demonstrable evidence of brain damage.

The damage to the brain may be generalized, affecting all aspects of cognitive functioning relatively equally, as in Down's syndrome, or it may affect parts of the brain responsible for the control of emotion, language function, activity and so on, relatively more than others. If this is the case, behaviour disturbance is more likely to be present. Furthermore the brain damage may cause impairment in a particular function. In this case its effect on behaviour will depend not only to the extent and the part of brain involved but also the stage of development at which the damage occurred and the degree to which other parts of the brain have been able to compensate. Thus recovery from head injury in young children may be more complete than from a similar injury occurring later in life.

Damage to the brain may also cause disturbance to other healthy parts of the brain if the damaged part is malfunctioning, rather than not functioning at all. This is seen most clearly when the damaged part of the brain is electrically active, as in some forms of partial epilepsy, where discharges arising from the damaged part spread to involve other parts of the brain. A striking example occurs in some cases of infantile hemiplegia where damage to one side of the brain has caused paralysis of the opposite arm, leg and side of the face. This is often associated with epilepsy and severe behaviour disturbance, with aggression and overactivity due to the spread of electrical disturbance from the damaged hemisphere to the healthy one. A similar mechanism also accounts in part for the considerable increase in behaviour disturbance seen in people with temporal lobe or psychomotor epilepsy. Often, the behaviourally disruptive effects stem less from the brain lesion itself, than from the effect of the lesion upon the remaining intact nervous system.

Brain damage is only one of a number of factors causing behavioural disturbance in the mentally retarded. Social factors, such as rejection by adults and peers, play an important part in causing emotional disturbance in retarded children. This relationship is complex because rejection may affect the child's emotional disturbance and children may be rejected equally because of their undesirable behavioural and temperamental characteristics.

It is now known that normal children differ, from the first few months of life, in temperamental factors such as poor adaptability to new situations, a high intensity of emotional response, marked irregularity of physiological functioning and activity level. These temperamental differences have been shown to be important in causing behavioural disorders in children of normal intelligence, and it seems likely that they are at least as important, if not more important, in retarded children.

It is the interaction of temperamental and environmental factors which leads to the particular style of adult environmental adaptation which we call personality. This is in part inherited as a result of genetic factors, and in part the result of experience and the influence of psychological and biological factors from the earliest stages of intrauterine development. This also explains why, in adult life, the mentally handicapped tend to show immature personality characteristics, often more typical of normal adolescents or younger children.

Intellectually retarded children are adversely affected by the same kinds of family and social stress in the community as other children, and parental instability, unsatisfactory discipline and family discord all lead to behavioural disturbance. A number of retarded children are cared for over long periods in institutions, and emotional disturbance may stem in these children from the ill effects of poor-quality institutional care. These effects are not invariable and depend to a large extent on the quality of care provided. Children may spend long periods in institutions in early childhood and yet develop normally, providing the environment is sufficiently stimulating and there is an opportunity to develop lasting relationships with other people. Nowadays when fewer children with less severe handicaps are admitted to institutional care, it is likely that behaviour disturbance is more frequently the cause rather than the result of institutionalization.

Emotional immaturity, language disorder and educational failure may also play a part in causing behavioural disturbance in people with mental handicap, but on the whole it may be concluded that organic cerebral dysfunction and temperamental factors are more important in the severely retarded, while psychosocial factors predominate in all the mildly retarded.

TYPES OF BEHAVIOUR DISORDER

As described in Chapter 6, recognizable psychotic illness of an adult type, e.g. manic depressive psychosis and schizophrenia, are a relatively uncommon cause of admission to hospital, together accounting for not more than about 6% of all hospital admissions. This may in part be due to the difficulty in diagnosis of conditions which depend, for their identification, so much on intact language functioning (Corbett, 1979). If cases of childhood psychosis persisting in adults with mental retardation are included, the prevalence of major mental illness in adults with mental retardation will rise; this accounts for the higher figure given by some authors (e.g. Tibbits, 1978).

Apart from these relatively uncommon illnesses, the full range of disorders seen in people of normal intelligence are also seen in the mentally handicapped. Thus neurotic disorders, with predominant anxiety, depression, phobias and sleep difficulty, are seen in children who are faced with a situation with which they are unable to cope, and undiagnosed mild mental retardation may be a cause of school phobia which will be most effectively managed by placing the child in a more appropriate educational setting.

Antisocial conduct, with aggression, stealing or destructive behaviour, will be modified by the child's ability to manifest the symptoms. Truancy from school, and stealing from outside the home, may be replaced in the more severely retarded child by wandering from home and a failure to learn the meaning of personal property at school or at home.

Although these types of behaviour disorders are somewhat increased in children with mental handicap a particular increase is seen in conditions involving the child's level of motor activity, the so-called hyperkinetic syndrome, and in symptoms of childhood psychosis or autism. In both these conditions many of the behavioural symptoms are related to a marked discrepancy between the child's gross motor skills and an inability to use language to mediate behaviour, communicate with others and engage in self-initiated play or other activities.

In addition to these more clearly defined syndromes, or constellations of symptoms, relatively isolated behaviour problems such as severe repetitive or stereotyped behaviour, which may be associated with self-injury; pica, involving the repeated ingestion of substances normally regarded as inedible; habitual regurgitation or vomiting may be sufficiently handicapping in day-to-day life to require treatment.

There are many forms of medical treatment which may be indicated in the mentally handicapped. Considerable skill may be required in the diagnosis of underlying physical illness which may be indirectly affecting behaviour in a person who has difficulty describing his symptoms or feelings. Among the most important of the conditions requiring treatment are intercurrent infection, other causes of pain, discomfort and epilepsy (Corbett, 1976; Pond and Corbett, 1979).

In this short account emphasis will however be given to medication given in order to directly affect behaviour.

PSYCHOTROPIC MEDICATION

Useful reviews of our present state of knowledge of drug-use in treating behaviour disorders in mentally handicapped people have been published by Sprague and Werry (1971), Freeman (1970), Lipton *et al.* (1977) and Heaton-Ward (1977), while a useful practical guide for parents and those responsible for the care of the mentally handicapped has recently been written by Freeman (1978).

The results of treating behaviour disorders with drugs alone tend to be disappointing in the long term, although there may be an initial response. Medical treatment should always be seen as part of a planned programme of management.

A period of initial response, whether it is caused by a temporary change in attitude on the part of parents or staff, or whether it is a genuine pharmacological effect, provides the opportunity to put the planned programme of behaviour management into effect (Brady, 1971).

Thus the control of hyperactivity may allow a child to settle and attend sufficiently to implement a programme aimed at shaping up occupational skills, or enable the child to be engaged in a programme of language training. Similarly medication given to reduce anxiety can be a powerful adjuvant to programmes of systematic desensitization in the case of specific phobias.

CLASSIFICATION OF PSYCHOTROPIC DRUGS

A. Major Tranquillizers

Phenothiazines such as chlorpromazine, thioridazine and pericyazine reduce anxiety and agitation and are probably the most widely used in the treatment of overactivity and a variety of other difficult behaviours (Lipman, 1970). It is often found that retarded people showing psychotic symptoms require larger doses of this and other drugs than does the normal child. Inadequate doses may exacerbate the behavioural symptoms and make the child more irritable, while large doses are prone to produce side-effects such as oversedation, impairment of learning and extrapyramidal effects including tremor and rigidity. Recent evidence suggests that the optimum therapeutic effect may only be achieved over quite a narrow range of blood levels, as is the case with anticonvulsants. At the present time, this technique is only available on an experimental basis for a few psychotropic drugs such as thioridazine. Extrapyramidal and other side-effects such as jaundice, blood dyscrasias and photosensitivity seem to be based on individual sensitivity.

Photosensitivity may be avoided by using thioridazine or pericyazine rather than chlorpromazine. Pericyazine, which can be given in a single daily dose at night-time, may avoid the sedative effects of other phenothiazines.

Piperazine derivatives such as trifluoperazine and perphenazine are less sedative in their action and may be particularly helpful in anxious patients where attempts to interrupt ritualistic behaviour result in temper-outbursts and distress. Although on the whole freer from side-effects, these drugs may cause acute dystonia in sensitive subjects and concomitant administration of anti-parkinsonian drugs is usually necessary.

In recent years the use of butyrophenone derivatives, such as haloperidol, in the mentally retarded has increased. In small doses this drug has the advantage of being given in drops in a colourless concentrate which may be helpful where there are difficulties over administration of drugs by mouth. This drug also may cause acute dystonia, but again this seems to be a matter of individual sensitivity. Occasionally patients become irritable and depressed; if this happens the drug should be withdrawn. Recently larger doses of haloperidol given by injection have replaced parenteral chlorpromazine or paraldehyde as a safe and more effective method of controlling outbursts of disturbed behaviour, including an extreme bout of agitation or aggression.

B.   Minor Tranquillizers

Drugs such as diazepam chlordiazepoxide, clorazepate, oxazepam or hydroxyzine are used mainly in the control of anxiety and have a limited place as an adjuvant to programmes of behavioural management in the mentally retarded. If given in the absence of such an effective environmental programme there is evidence that they may increase agitation and release aggression in some cases.

C.   Antidepressants

These are rarely indicated in the treatment of behavioural disturbance in retarded children unless there is clear-cut evidence of super-added affective illness. Imipramine derivatives may however be helpful when given at night in some cases of nocturnal enuresis when the child has reached a stage when this is developmentally inappropriate.

D.   Stimulant Drugs

Drugs such as amphetamine or methylphenidate are rarely as effective in controlling hyperactivity as they are in carefully selected cases of the hyperkinetic syndrome in children of normal intelligence. They may, however, occasionally be indicated.

E. Barbiturates

These are also usually ineffective in the control of overactive aggressive behaviour and, in subjects with brain damage, may paradoxically increase overactivity and irritability. This particularly applies to the use of phenobarbitone and also primidone in the treatment of epilepsy in such patients. This response, however, seems to be a matter of individual sensitivity. In view of their effectiveness as anticonvulsants these drugs may occasionally be indicated on a trial basis.

F. Hypnotic and other Sedative Drugs

Chloral hydrate, nitrazepam and flurazepam are probably most effective where adequate behavioural and environmental manipulation has failed to help with persistent sleep disturbance; again care must be taken to ensure that this is part of a planned intervention to restore a biologically more appropriate sleep pattern and does not lead to hangover effects, irritability and sedation by day.

G. Lithium Carbonate

A number of studies suggest that lithium may be effective where there is a periodic or cyclical quality to the patient's behaviour disturbance and where this is associated with changes in affect, although claims of a more sustained effect on aggressive or impulsive behaviour have been less effectively substantiated (Cambell, 1975).

H. Anticonvulsant Drugs

These are rarely indicated in the treatment of behavioural disorders unless there is clinical or electroencephalographic evidence of epilepsy. In this case it is essential that the drug administration is carefully monitored by the estimation of blood levels. Generally speaking it is preferable to. use anticonvulsants such as carbamazepine or sodium valproate, with the least side-effects, and where possible to use a single drug. Sulthiame, although probably an ineffective anticonvulsant on its own, may be effective in combination with other anticonvulsants in the control of hyperactivity in some instances.

I.   General Principles underlying Psychotropic Drug
     Administration in the Mentally Handicapped

(a) Psychotropic drugs should not generally be given in the absence of an adequate environmental programme for management of the individual's behaviour.
(b) Individual differences in metabolism and reaction are considerable and may be more marked in subjects with brain damage. Wherever possible an individualized trial of the sort described by Shapiro (1966) should be carried out before a drug is used routinely.
(c) There are very few instances in which specific drugs seem to be effective in controlling individual symptoms; all psychotropic drugs which are in common usage have general effects. It has, for example, been suggested that thioridazine is particularly effective in controlling stereotyped behaviour, but it is one of the few drugs which has been subjected to an adequate controlled trial in this condition. Possible exceptions to this rule are the uses of 5-hydroxytryptophan and carbidopa to control self-injurious behaviour in the Lesch–Nyhan syndrome (a rare inborn error of uric acid metabolism) (Nyhan, 1976) and baclofen, also in the management of self-injury in other patients (Primrose, 1979). The specificity and long-term effects of these forms of medication remain to be established.
(d) Most psychotropic drugs have an immediate short-term effect, but tolerance often develops and the tendency to progressively increase drug dose, or add an alternative drug, in these circumstances without withdrawal of the previous medication should be avoided if possible. It should be remembered that many drugs given in combination tend to interact.
(e) Generally speaking, administration of drugs should be started at a low dose and gradually increased until an optimum effect is achieved. Similarly drugs should be withdrawn gradually where possible, as there is evidence that emergent dystonic

MEDICAL TREATMENT OF BEHAVIOUR PROBLEMS

Table 4.1 Brief classification of psychotropic drugs

A. *Major tranquillizers* (also called 'antipsychotic' or 'neuroleptic' drugs) reduce anxiety, agitation, hallucinations and delusions. They are most useful in the major psychoses of adult life but also for some other problems.
    Examples are: chlorpromazine (Largactil); thioridazine (Melleril); pericyazine (Neulactil); haloperidol (Serenace, Haldol); trifluoperazine (Stelazine); fluphenazine (Modecate); pimozide (Orap).

    Side-effects include: sleepiness, depression, low blood pressure, an increase in seizures or sometimes seizures in someone who has never had any, constipation, weight gain and abnormal movements. Rarely: eye and liver changes, skin rashes and sensitivity to sunlight.

B. *Minor tranquillizers* have limited use, in mentally retarded people, in reducing anxiety and treating some seizure disorders.

    Examples are: diazepam (Valium); chlordiazepoxide (Librium); clorazepate (Tranxene).

    Side-effects include: drowsiness and increased agitation.

C. *Antidepressants* are used to elevate mood and reduce bedwetting.

    Examples are: imipramine (Tofranil); amitriptyline (tryptizol).

    Side-effects include: changes in heart function, dry mouth, urinary retention and seizures.

D. *Stimulants* increase activity of part of the nervous system.

    Examples are: methylphenidate (Ritalin); dextroamphetamine (Dexedrine).

    Side-effects include: insomnia, loss of appetite, over-excitability and tearfulness.

E. *Sedatives* may be used to slow an individual down or to induce sleep. They may impair co-ordination and intellectual functions.

    Examples are: barbiturates; chloral hydrate; nitrazepam (Mogadon); flurazepam (Dalmane).

    Side-effects include: stomach upset, irritability and hangover.

F. *Anti-parkinsonian drugs* are used to counteract the nervous system side-effects of other psychoactive drugs, especially the major tranquillizers.

    Examples are: benztropine (Cogentin); benzhexol (Artane).

    Side-effects include: dry mouth, constipation, depression, weakness, nausea, urinary retention.

effects may be precipitated both with major and minor tranquillizers in handicapped people (Poliezos, *et al.*, 1973).

(f) Changes in drug effectiveness may occur with age, and careful monitoring, although essential at all times, is particularly necessary at certain stages of development; e.g. during the adolescent growth spurt.

In conclusion it may be stated that the ideal psychotropic drug for helping the person with mental retardation with severely disturbed behaviour does not exist. In view of the multiplicity of actions, and what is known of the metabolism of most classes of psychotropic drugs, together with the multiplicity and interaction of the many factors usually involved in causing behaviour disturbance, it is unlikely that this situation will be remedied in the near future.

In the meantime judicious drug use, following clinical trials in individual cases and careful monitoring, may be a crucial adjuvant to the implementation of an adequate programme of behavioural environmental management in dealing with severely handicapping behaviour problems in the mentally handicapped.

References

Brady, J. P. (1971). Drugs in behaviour therapy. In Masserman, J. M. (ed.) *Current Psychiatric Therapies*. Vol. II. (New York: Grune & Stratton)

Cambell, M., Fish, B., Korein, J., Shapiro, T., Collins, P. and Koh, R. C., (1972). Lithium and chlorpromazine. A controlled crossover study of hyperactive severely disturbed young children. *J. Autism Child. Schizophr.*, 2, 234

Corbett, J. A. (1976). Medical man gement. In Wing, L. (ed.) *Early Childhood Autism*. 2nd Edn. (Oxf rd: Pergamon)

Corbett, J. A. (1977). Mental retardatic 1 – psychiatric aspects. In Rutter, M. and Hersov, L. (eds.) *Child Psychiatry*. (Oxford: Blackwell)

Corbett, J. A. (1979). Psychiatric morbidity in mental retardation. In James, F. E. and Snaith, R. P. (eds.) *Psychiatric Aspects of Mental Handicap.* (London: Gaskell)

Freeman, R. D. (1970). Psychopharmacology and the retarded child. In Menolascino, F. J. (ed.) *Psychiatric Approaches to Mental Retardation.* (New York: Basic Books)

Freeman, R. D. (1978). *The Use of Drugs to Modify Behaviour in Retarded Persons: A Practical Guide for Parents and Advocates*. Monograph Supplement to *Mental Retardation*. (Ontario: Canadian Association for the Mentally Retarded)

Heaton-Ward, W. A. (1977). The drug treatment of mentally handicapped patients in hospital. In Mittler, P. (ed.) *Research to Practice in Mental Retardation. Vol. III. Biomedical Aspects.* 1 ASSMD (Lancaster: MTP Press)

Lipman, R. S. (1970). The use of psychopharmacological agents in residential facilities for the retarded. In Gaull, G. E. (ed.) *Biology of Brain Dysfunction.* 1. (New York: Plenum Press)

Lipton, M. A., Nemeroff, C. B., Bissette, G. and Prange, A. J. Jr. (1977). The role of drugs in the prevention and treatment of mental retardation. In Mittler, P. (ed.) *Research to Practice in Mental Retardation. Vol. III. Biomedical Aspects.* 1 ASSMD (Lancaster: MTP Press)

Nyhan, W. L. (1976). Behaviour in the Lesch–Nyhan syndrome. *J. Autism Child. Schizophr.,* 6, 235

Poliezos, P., Engelhardt, D. M., Hoffman, S. P. and Waizer, J. (1973). Neurological consequences of psychotropic drug withdrawal in schizophrenic children. *J. Autism Child. Schizophr.,* 6, 247

Pond, D. A. and Corbett, J. A. (1979). Epilepsy. In James, F. E. and Snaith, R. P. (eds.) *Psychiatric Aspects of Mental Handicap.* (London: Gaskell)

Primrose, D. (1979). Baclofen in the treatment of self-injurious behaviour. Paper read at Congress of ASSMD, Jerusalem.

Rutter, M. (1971). Psychiatry. In Wortis, J. (ed.) *Mental Retardation. Vol. III. An Annual Review.* (New York: Grune & Stratton)

Sprague, R. L. and Werry, J. S. (1971). Methodology of pharmacological studies with the retarded. In Ellis, N. R. (ed.) *International Review of Research in Mental Retardation.* Vol. 5. (New York: Academic Press)

5

THE BEHAVIOURAL APPROACH

C. Williams

INTRODUCTION

Throughout history the mentally handicapped have been dealt with according to the prevailing view of the time. They have been regarded as objects of reverence and worship, scorn and derision, fear and revulsion, pity and charity, or simply in need of care and protection. More recently, with the rising interest in the rights of the handicapped as persons, many services have been developed with the aim of enabling mentally handicapped people to live as independently as possible in a normal environment.

The behavioural approach is one of several that can influence the achievement of such an aim. Its great strength lies in its clear objectives and methodology and built-in evaluative and monitoring procedures. These allow the careworker to answer the questions – where am I going? – how will I get there? – and how will I know when I have arrived? It is essentially a method of teaching based upon the application of principles derived from the theory known as operant learning and largely derived from the work of Skinner (1974) and his colleagues.

One of the most crucial aspects in the theoretical background is its philosophy regarding the causes or determinants of behaviour. This forms the context within which actual programmes of teaching or training can be developed.

43

THE PHILOSOPHY OF THE BEHAVIOURAL APPROACH

In attempting to find reasons why people do things, we frequently refer to personality or emotional state; or in discussing how people learn to do things we refer to intelligence and motivation. None of these 'explanations' – emotion, personality, intelligence, motivation – is directly observable and we can only infer for instance, that Mary bites other children because of her aggressive personality, or that John has tantrums because of his frustration.

When these explanations are examined we find they are incomplete. To say that Mary bites because of her aggressive personality invites the question – 'how do we know she has an aggressive personality?', to which the answer is – because she bites other people. Similarly, to say that John has tantrums because he is frustrated begs the question – 'how do we know he is frustrated?', to which we reply – because he has tantrums. These traditional explanations in fact tell us nothing more about the behaviour than we already know. We are simply equating biting with aggression and tantrums with frustration. In other words this approach does little more than provide a sophisticated description that masquerades as an explanation.

One very common statement is that 'John does not learn because he is mentally handicapped', often as an explanation for his failure. It begs the question – how do we know he is mentally handicapped? To this we say – because he does not learn! This last example is all the more tragic because it suggests that any failure to learn on John's part is due to his mental handicap alone. It is important to recognize that the term mental handicap does *not* explain his failure to learn, it only renames the observation derived from his behaviour, or lack of it. The behavioural approach suggests that to use indefinable processes as explanations is unnecessary and misleading. The approach is directly concerned with behaviour; with what people actually do or say. Probably the best way of deciding whether or not you are actually dealing with behaviour is to see if you can record it when it occurs – in other words you cannot record frustration as a behaviour, but you can record face-slapping and the circumstances of its occurrence as observable events.

44

THE FOUR STAGES OF BEHAVIOURAL STRATEGY

The principle of recording brings us to the strategy used in implementing behavioural training programmes. This may be broken down into four stages, each of which is important in planning programmes.

STAGE ONE: ASSESSMENT

Assessment is the crucial first stage as it tells us which aspects of the person's behaviour are immediately important; which need a longer-term view; and, most important, where to start.

There are basically two classes of behaviour in which we are interested. One class refers to those skills that have *not* been learned but which he might have been expected to acquire at his age. We know for instance that most children by the age of 6 years can wash, dress, feed and toilet themselves relatively independently. If you assess a 10-year-old child *without physical handicap* and he is unable to perform these self-care skills you would be likely to say that he was retarded in his development – or that he had *deficits* in his repertoire of skills. However, you would not say this if the child was only 2 years old; nor would you say it if you assessed his ability to speak Russian. Although he might not have that skill in his repertoire you would not consider it an important deficit – unless of course he was Russian. It is important to appreciate that skills are only crucial if their absence is handicapping a person in his ability to live independently. The acquiring of non-crucial skills – for instance, translating classical Greek – is only of value once the basic personal and social skills have been acquired.

Methods and Forms used in Assessment

The skills assessed must therefore be crucial to independence and related to the developmental progress of the individual. To assess the repertoire of skills or abilities, and from that to deduce relevant deficit areas for teaching, we need to use some form of assessment scale. You can develop your own scale, but it is much better to use standard and well-tested scales developed by people involved in devising such instruments, based upon normal psychological and behavioural development. Assessment scales may also use a task-analysis approach where relevant target behaviours are chosen and are broken down into their component parts in sequence. This can then form the basis of a teaching programme and also indicate the starting point of the programme. Another type of assessment scale compares the client with an average group of persons of the same age and tells you whether or not he is above, below or the same as this 'normal' group. The first two kinds of assessment are more useful for programme planning.

Examples of these assessment forms are many, and details are given in the bibliography. Amongst the most commonly used are the following:

> Vineland Social Maturity Scale (Doll).
> Progress Assessment Charts (Gunsberg).
> Adaptive Behaviour Scales (American Association on Mental Deficiency).
> Social Training Achievement Records (Williams).
> Behaviour Checklist (Perkins, Capie and Taylor).
> Parental Involvement Project (Cunningham and Jeffree).
> Fairview Self-Help Scale.
> Behaviour Assessment Battery (Kiernan and Jones).

You should be able to find one of these to suit your own particular needs. It is better to use one of them consistently so that you can check on results over a period of time. They will all provide a profile of skills from which you can infer the deficits which become the goals of your initial training programmes.

The other group of behaviours includes those already present but which are considered to be inappropriate. This covers behaviours such as self-injury and aggressive acts to others, or can be even more bizarre, like clothes tearing and faeces smearing. These undesirable activities can be considered to have been learned; they are therefore capable of being unlearned or of having some other more acceptable behaviour take their place.

The assessment of bizarre, inappropriate or deviant behaviour is different from that of assessing skills related to competency. To start with, a simple diary should be kept of every occurrence of deviant behaviour. This method is called *event recording* and

would be useful for such activities as window breaking or tantrums, when they do not happen too frequently.

Another way of observing and recording behaviour already
present is to use a process called *time sampling*. Here you can
either record what a person is doing at a given point in time (for
instance, writing down what he is doing at 5-minute intervals
depending on the frequency of the behaviour throughout the day).
A timer may be used to give a signal at the time interval chosen. At
this point the observer would note down the activity of the person
being observed. Another method is to write down all that the
person does for an interval of, say, 1 minute, every 30 minutes. This
is known as *interval recording*.

These methods are appropriate for different forms of
behaviour, and choice will depend on nature and frequency of
occurrence. After a period of time you will have built up a
comprehensive picture of the types of deviant behaviour present,
and of their frequency.

Summary

Assessment provides information both on the competence of a
person and on his deviant behaviours (see Table 5.1).

Table 5.1 Recording behaviour

Type of behaviour	Methods of assessment and recording
Assets, skills, competences	Developmental checklists, skill checklists, training records, standardized tests
Deviant, inappropriate, disruptive, bizarre behaviours	Time sampling, event recording, interval recording

STAGE TWO: INTERPRETATION

Once the assessment of the individual is completed priorities can
be decided: does he need to learn new skills or does he need to
unlearn some of the skills he already has; or should the programme
be a combination of both? Before we can start, however, we have
to make some informed interpretation or hypothesis, from our

47

observations. Why is the individual unable to use a knife and fork? Why can he not put all of his clothes on yet? Why does he have tantrums at meal times? We have to make interpretations of each of these behaviours. In other words we need to explore the determinants or *causes* of his behaviour.

Determinants of Behaviour

Explanations of behaviour are varied: 'that's the way we are – it's in our blood – it's in our personality – it's part of inner motivation *or* of our instincts'. However, looking closely at these reasons, especially if you wish to know how to change behaviour, you will find they are not very helpful. They do not give ideas for change. You can only change or modify the behaviour of a person (or yourself) if you can both *identify* and *manipulate* the reasons or causes of that person's behaviour. Sometimes you can identify the causes but cannot manipulate them; sometimes you may be manipulating the causes but fail to identify them. Most times, however, we attempt neither to identify nor to manipulate the causes.

There are two main sources for variation in the behaviour of a person. The first comes from his physical or biological make up and can be said to be determined largely by his *heredity* – what he inherited from his parents. The second comes from the experiences he has – his *environment* and what has happened to him. These two sources interact to produce the behaviour we see in people. There may well be other causes; some people would argue strongly that there were; but until they can be clearly identified and manipulated they are not much help to us in assisting handicapped people to become independent and more acceptable to society.

Causes

This list shows some of the causes:

1. *Heredity*. The variation due to the action and influence of our genetic make-up contributes to our physical appearance and probably also the rate or efficiency with which we can learn (usually referred to as our intelligence).

2. *Environmental.* It is important to recognize that our behaviour is influenced by two forms of environment: an internal environment within ourselves, and the one we normally associate with the word environment – namely the world outside, our surroundings; both people and things. Both of these can influence our behaviour either separately or interactively.

Internal

(a) *Changes in anatomy, physiology and metabolism (biochemical events).* Changes in our body resulting in restricted movement (motor handicap) and changes in our body's way of working when we experience changes in our heart rate, our breathing, our digestive system, can all influence our behaviour. We feel afraid or excited, hungry or thirsty or become increasingly aware of a full bladder. Each of these changes in the body can influence or determine our behaviour. The use of medication to change the behaviour of people is an example of modifying some of the body's biochemical or internal workings which in turn influence behaviour. Medication can, therefore, be seen as a process of modifying behaviour. However, it only has an effect on behaviour already present in a person. No medication has yet been invented that will *teach* you anything new, although it may assist you to learn by removing or reducing reactions or states which decrease your efficiency.

(b) *Thoughts (cognitive events).* Through our experience with the outside world and with increased knowledge of how we interact with it we build up a conceptual representation of the world – in most cases expressed in language form. We generally think in words; some people think in actions or symbols; it depends upon your previous experience and learning. This inner cognitive environment can also influence how we behave. The development of cognitive behaviour therapy is an example of how changes in behaviour can be brought about by assisting people to make changes in the way they think about or conceptualize their behaviour. Unfortunately, with many mentally handicapped persons their language ability is not

49

developed to the extent where this form of behaviour modification would be the method of first choice.

External

(a) *Discriminative stimuli (setting events)*. The world about us impinges on us continuously through our hearing, sight, touch, smell and taste. Through our experience with these stimuli we come to learn different ways of reacting to them. We learn to stop when we see a red light, to run when we see our bus leaving or to say 'thank you' when given a sweet. These circumstances are the same for the mentally handicapped and they can quickly learn, for instance, the settings in which it is worthwhile having a tantrum. They can learn that in some settings talking has no effect on the environment. They can come to learn that a greater effect can be achieved by urinating on the carpet rather than in the lavatory. All of these acts are influenced by the discriminative stimuli or signals received from outside. In a way they inform us of the most effective time and place to produce a behaviour to get the most effect. If a person has only a restricted repertoire of behaviours then stereotyped or similar responses are likely in response to the environment. The wider the repertoire is, the greater is the adaptability to environmental change. Therefore, teaching new and varied skills to the mentally handicapped should be more beneficial to them than concentrating on the removal of inappropriate or deviant behaviour. It is also true that the more able or competent a person is the more will strange behaviour be tolerated in him by others.

3. *Physical and historical influences on behaviour*. There are two other areas which provide possible explanations for our behaviour: one is our physical make-up and the other is the influence of past experience.

(a) *Physical determinants*. The basic size and shape of a person can influence his behaviour. Altering a person's weight for instance can be very effective in changing behaviour! In the handicapped, the major physical determinants are usually because of deficiencies of input and/or output.

Input dysfunctions: these may occur when stimuli from the outside world either are not received at all or are incorrectly received or interpreted by the person. This may be due to defect in the hearing system or the visual system or both. These defects can occur at any level in those systems and have a marked effect on the learning ability of the individual. Procedures to compensate for minor dysfunctions are essential – amplifiers for the partially hearing, and spectacles for the visually handicapped. It is crucial that assessment of the sensory capacity of the handicapped is carried out as early as possible because, although they react to the defect with incorrect, unacceptable or inappropriate behaviour, they may not be able to indicate the defect themselves.

Output dysfunctions: these usually occur when the individual has difficulty either in controlling or initiating movements of his body. He may suffer from a form of cerebral palsy, for instance, which results in rigidity of his limbs or an inability to control his movements.

(b) *Historical determinants.* Clearly our present behaviour is very much influenced by our past experiences. It is shaped by the effects which our actions have had in the past. We can often see in the history of an individual how it was he came to behave the way he does now. It is also clearly illogical to attempt to explain behaviour by referring to future events since, by definition, those events have not yet occurred and cannot therefore influence present behaviour. For instance, we do not go to a restaurant for the first time because we will be given a meal there, but because we have previously learned that restaurants provide meals and therefore there is a high probability that this will be repeated. This involved two separate processes – the first is the actual experience and the second is the person's ability to learn from it and remember it for future reference. By carefully looking into the history of a behaviour problem you may find reasons for its existence. Unfortunately, you cannot modify or remove these if they

51

occurred in the past. They may even no longer be influencing the present behaviour of the person. Hence, although historical events are important in *explaining* behaviour they frequently play little part in the third stage of behaviour modification, that of *intervention*.

(c) *Effects of antecedent and consequential events.* Before we come to formulating or putting programmes into practice, there are further events that influence behaviour. These are the events which *antecede* or come before the behaviour, and those events which *follow* its occurrence or form the consequences of the behaviour.

From many experimental studies and from our own experience, we can see that the consequences of behaviour can have one of two main effects. They can make it *more likely* that we will repeat the action in the future under the same circumstances or, alternatively, make it *less likely* that the action will be repeated in the future under the same circumstances.

Various terms are used in behaviour modification to describe the more specific effects of these situations on behaviour. In the first instance the behaviour is *strengthened* or *reinforced*; in the second it is said that the behaviour is *weakened* or *punished*.

A third effect that can be observed is when a behaviour that has been strengthened or reinforced in the past is no longer followed by the event that had been functioning as a reinforcer. This also has the effect of *weakening* the behaviour, but the process in this case is known as *extinction*.

A fourth effect that can also occur is when a behaviour is followed by the removal of an event that can potentially function as a punisher. This also has the effect of *strengthening* or *reinforcing* that behaviour. This process is known as *negative reinforcement*.

A fifth effect occurs when a behaviour is followed by the *removal* of an event that can potentially function as a reinforcer. This has the effect of *weakening* or *punishing* that behaviour. This process could be referred to as negative punishment but is more usually known as *response cost*.

All of this might sound complicated, and in real life it can, indeed, become very complex. There are times when a combination or interaction of causes and effects operate simultaneously. A simplistic view of behaviour modification, which only suggests rewards and punishments, fails to provide an adequate analysis of the behaviour and is unlikely to be successful or lasting in its effect. Table 5.2 summarizes the descriptions given above; the nature of the consequences; the term by which the process is usually known and the effect it has on the behaviour it follows. This model can be further summarized by considering the two main classes of events that can influence behaviour: setting events and consequating

Table 5.2 Summary of events and descriptions of effects

Consequating event	Known as	Effect on behaviour
Presentation of a reinforcer	Positive reinforcement	Strengthen
Presentation of a punisher	Punishment	Weaken
Cessation of reinforcement	Extinction	Weaken
Removal of punishing event	Negative reinforcement	Strengthen
Removal of reinforcing event	Response cost	Weaken

events. The setting events are referred to as the antecedents of the behaviour as they come *before* the behaviour occurs, and the consequating events come *after* the behaviour as consequences. Hence the model can be simply written as:

$$A \longrightarrow B \longrightarrow C$$
$$\text{(Antecedents)} \quad \text{(Behaviour)} \quad \text{(Consequences)}$$

By identifying both the antecedents and consequences of the behaviour a programme of intervention can be drawn up.

STAGE THREE: INTERVENTION

Two main areas of behaviour will concern us here: those which we have decided from our assessment need to be taught as short-term goals leading towards normality and independence, and those which we have decided from our observations need eliminating as interfering with eventual normality and independence. In other words our plan of intervention will be to increase competence and to decrease deviance, leading to an increased acceptance by society.

Increasing Competence

From our initial assessment we will know at what point to start teaching. It is of little use to teach reading and writing to someone who is not yet able to control his bowels or use a knife and fork independently. The aim of teaching new skills to mentally handicapped people is to build upon their assets; to start with what they can already do and develop those skills whilst slowly introducing new skills by *prompting* or *modelling*.

Prompting

All too often we expect mentally handicapped people to understand immediately what it is we want them to do. We frequently use language that is too complex, and instructions that are too long. It is something like giving people instructions in a foreign language so that they cannot comply, not because of being uncooperative, or not in the mood, or mentally handicapped, but because they do not have the prerequisite skill to understand the instruction. We know that we can make ourselves understood by using gestures, and this is one way of indicating to handicapped people what is wanted of them. You can point, or beckon, or show them what you want; if that does not work, then you can take their hands in yours and guide them through the desired actions. This manual guidance or physical prompting procedure is very helpful when teaching manipulative skills like self-feeding or assembly tasks. Always remember to reinforce even these assisted steps. It is these small successes that will lead on to more complex tasks. You might find that a range of reinforcers will work, but generally praise and touch will be effective. If not, then look for something else that your student or trainee will work for – it might even be a taste of ice-cream or small pieces of chocolate.

Modelling

This procedure relies upon your having taught your student or trainee how to imitate your actions. You can do this using the prompt-and-reinforcement method. Once he can reliably copy what you do when you ask him, you can short-circuit much of the prompting merely by saying 'John, do this' and then demonstrating the whole action. This would be useful, for instance, in self-help skills training when teaching him how to wash his hands and face, or more complex tasks in education or work settings, which may need to be broken down into simpler steps each of which is rewarded or reinforced in the initial period of teaching.

Rules in Teaching

There are many examples of using techniques derived from the behavioural approach to teach new skills. They rely on a number of important rules:

> break the task down into small steps;
> teach these steps one at a time;
> reinforce the learning of each new step;
> try and link the learning of a new step with a step already learned;
> try and make the task itself rewarding;
> bring the completion of the entire task into the everyday activity of the individual in order not to have to use some artificial or unnatural means to maintain the skill;
> teach only relevant tasks.

The books mentioned in the bibliography contain many such examples and are recommended to the reader for further details of specific teaching programmes.

Decreasing Deviant and Unacceptable Behaviour

For a number of years, when behaviour modification was beginning to have an impact in the care of the mentally handicapped, it appeared as though its main purpose was to assist in the removal of those behaviours that were either personally damaging: self-injury and such-like; or else were distressing to others: tantrums, excessive overactivity, stripping off clothes and so on. Some very effective methods were reported; and dramatic changes, for instance from severe self-mutilation and isolation to developing more socially acceptable behaviours, were reported. However, many of these reports used fairly drastic techniques of *punishment* or of *response cost* where the consequences of the unacceptable deviant behaviours were designed to be aversive, with little consideration being given to providing more acceptable alternatives. This was often because the therapists had only dealt superficially with the behaviour in isolation and had not analysed its function within the person's own total life.

Elimination of Identifiable Causes

It must not be forgotten that some disturbed or deviant behaviours may not have their origins in learning at all, but may be initiated for some physiological or clinical reason. Before using treatment techniques derived from behavioural principles it is important to check for and correct these causes where possible. Physical deformities that prevent certain movements, acute earache or toothache that may be the causative factor in head- or face-slapping are examples. This is even more essential when the person has no means of communicating his problem to you. Some forms of epilepsy may be associated with disturbed behaviour. In these circumstances, elimination of pain and/or control of the epilepsy is essential before the disturbed behaviour can be eliminated.

Analysis and Programming

Once these possible causes have been eliminated, then an intervention based upon a functional analysis of the behaviour can be implemented. In a functional analysis we ask the question 'What function or purpose does this behaviour have for the person?' The assumption is made that all behaviour has a reason, and functional analysis is aimed at finding out what it is in the person's environment that provides it, so that it can be altered to change the behaviour. Since a major component of the handicapped person's environment consists of behaviour of other people towards him, the reactions of these people form an important part of the analysis.

Example

Paul, a 12-year-old mentally handicapped child, had for a number of years developed a severe form of self-injury which consisted of slapping his head with his open palms; this was sufficient, if not attended to rapidly, to cause injury to his ears. Medication had not had any long-term benefit. Physical examination showed no reason for the behaviour. Following assessment and before intervention, two questions were asked:

1. Under what conditions did the behaviour occur; what were its setting and antecedents?
2. Were there reinforcers present?

It was found that he would head-bang only in the presence of people. When observed unobtrusively he ceased to do so, but would do so if anyone approached. It was also found that the most likely consequences were either that he would be picked up and cuddled, or given a biscuit or drink, or taken to the swing and pushed on it for a few minutes. Each of these interventions had the effect of stopping his self-injury.

Given this information we can begin to carry out a simple functional analysis. It is important to recognize, first of all, that there are at least two people involved: Paul *and* the person who intervenes. We have to account for the behaviour of both by the analysis. As far as the persons intervening are concerned we can see that the antecedents for their intervention include seeing Paul hitting his head; this caused them to approach Paul. It was likely that if Paul were not head-banging he would have been left alone. The sight of a mentally handicapped child indulging in self-injury is upsetting, and clearly any action that can stop it is likely to be found rewarding to the people around. This process of being rewarded or reinforced for the stopping of an aversive event has been referred to earlier as negative reinforcement. It has the function of making it more likely that the next time Paul hits his head, someone will again approach him and repeat the action previously found to have been effective in stopping the head-banging. In this case it was often a drink or a push on the swing.

From Paul's point of view it can be seen that the antecedent or setting for his self-injurious behaviour was the presence of another person, and also that the consequences functioned as positive reinforcement. It was therefore made more likely that next time he saw another person he would head-bang because, in the past, when he did so he was given a biscuit or cuddle or a push on the swing.

We can now see that we have described a 'behavioural circle' in which the behaviour of one person maintains that of another which in turn maintains the behaviour of the first person. Whilst Paul was reinforced by cuddles for head-banging, the person doing the cuddling was being reinforced by Paul, who stopped head-banging. This worked until the person could no longer continue cuddling Paul, or pushing him on the swing, or giving him biscuits. The problem behaviour remained and was in fact being strengthened by the very means being used to stop it. Although cessation of self-injury was achieved in the short term, it made it more likely to be repeated in the long run.

A longer-term view was developed: it was suggested that instead of dealing immediately with the head-banging we should consider that behaviour to be a form of 'communication'. It could be argued that Paul was using head-banging to 'ask for' a cuddle or a swing since he had *no other means of communication*. We therefore saw our task not as to how we could stop the head-banging; but how we could teach Paul an alternative method of asking. We chose a behaviour that was incompatible with head-banging; namely hand-clapping. You cannot clap your hands and hit your head at the same time. Paul would not clap his hands in the normal course of events and, even if he did, it was unlikely that people around him would have paid much attention as we might have assumed that he was happy and should be left alone. We have to use the teaching method of prompt-and-reinforce in order to enable Paul to learn first to clap his hands and second that clapping hands was as useful a behaviour as was head-banging to get his reward.

Method

Two people initially worked with Paul: one person to prompt

hand-clapping by using manual guidance; the second to reinforce it with cuddles, biscuits or drinks. Paul very quickly learned that hand-clapping led to exactly the same consequences as his earlier head-banging had done. Gradually we could afford to ignore attempts at head-banging because Paul had been *taught an alternative and more appropriate means of communication:* hand-clapping. Over time this hand-clapping can be 'shaped' into a wider range of non-vocal communication skills.

Principles Involved

The main principles involved in this example were:
    identification of the setting for the behaviour;
    identification of the consequences of the behaviour;
    establishing that the consequences are likely to be functioning as reinforcers;
    not to deny access to these reinforcers;
    not to punish the inappropriate behaviour;
but to teach an alternative behaviour to achieve the same ends or consequences;
and to build upon this alternative behaviour to increase the repertoire of more socially appropriate skills.

STAGE FOUR: EVALUATION

The final stage in the four-stage process of implementing behavioural programmes is the stage of evaluation. We need to know whether or not the programme actually worked. It is very easy to be hoodwinked into believing it was effective because of the effort put into its practice. The best method of evaluation is to repeat the steps taken at the start in the assessment and observation of the behaviour, and then to compare present results with previous ones.

Example: Toilet-training Programme

These principles can be applied to the development of a toilet-training programme, for instance.

1. Establish baseline measures of the child's behaviour: usually

done by ½-hourly checks of clothing throughout the day for about 2 weeks.
2. From the record find out the most likely times when the bladder and bowels are emptied, to decide on optimum toileting times.
3. Keep records of toileting performance throughout training – this might take the form shown in Table 5.3.

Table 5.3 Toilet performance record

Time	Mon.	Tues.	Wed.	Thurs.	Fri.	Sat.	Sun.
7.30	WSO	WUD	WU	WO	CUD	WO	WO
10.30	CU	CO	CO	CUD	CO	CUD	CU
12.30	CO	CU	CU	CO	WO	CO	CUD
3.30	WO	CU	WO	CO	WO	CU	CO
6.30	CU	CO	CU	CO	WO	CO	WO
9.30	WD	WSO	CUD	CU	WO	CU	CU

W – wet; S – soiled; C – clean and dry; U – urinated; D – defaecated; O – did nothing.

From this record we can see that the person was toileted six times each day. We can also see that some 45% of his total urinations (W and U) are recorded as occurring in his clothes (W) and some 55% are recorded as occurring when toileted (U). Similarly, some 22% of his total bowel movements (S and D) are recorded as soiling (S) whilst 78% are recorded as occurring when toileted (D). By keeping such a record, and plotting percentage points on a graph over time, a more accurate picture of change can be obtained than by trying to remember if any improvement has been shown since the previous review, perhaps 6 months ago.

Evaluation also enables the programme to be developed continuously. It is not appropriate to allow someone to remain at a particular task for long periods of time. There should be constant review, and a progressive plan of action produced, to continue the process of developing increased social competence and independence.

ETHICAL CONSIDERATIONS

In any programme of intervention there will be ethical implications requiring decisions. These relate to the methods and objectives of the programme. There will clearly be some methods of behaviour change that may be effective but which are of such a nature that the ethics of their use would be questionable. The means do not always justify the ends and, what is more important, there may be alternative means to achieving the same ends. The setting of objectives or goals creates a similar dilemma. Is the programme designed to develop the independence of the trainee or is it designed to make the work of the staff easier at the expense of the needs of the client? It can only be defensible if the aims of the programme are clearly to the benefit of the trainee. Decisions as to the appropriateness of objectives should be made by a multidisciplinary group of professionals, and parents wherever possible, through discussion by a properly constituted review team.

SUMMARY

A behaviour modification programme must be based on a knowledge of its philosophy coupled with a knowledge of relevant experimental work and study of the background; this enables a more effective functional analysis to be made of the problem behaviour and thus a more effective programme of teaching to be designed. The four-stage process – assessment; interpretation; intervention; evaluation, should not be short-circuited as it ensures an objective approach and a systematic review and examination of progress. In other words, this approach allows for methods to be developed for working with the most severely handicapped. Its methodology can be stated in clear terms which can be easily understood by all those connected with it.

PROCEDURAL GUIDELINES

The following procedural guidelines should help in all programme planning:

Complete an overall assessment to describe assets, deficits and excesses.

From this assessment *pinpoint realistic targets:* both long-term and short-term.

Record the baseline performance of the individual on the tasks to be taught – in other words, find out what he *can* do already and build from there.

Agree on programme steps – many of the tasks will have to be broken down into steps by the process of task analysis; this is best done by the training team who can then agree on the number, the size and the order of the steps in the task.

Use consequences that are effective as reinforcers – not all consequences may be reinforcing to everyone; the only way to find effective reinforcers is to test them out. Do they, in fact, increase or maintain the behaviour? The range of events that can function as reinforcers is very wide and might include, for any one individual, praise, sweets, physical contact, music, drinks and play. You have to find out what will work for each person you teach.

Record progress – keeping records can be tedious but it is the only effective way of seeing if the programme is working or not. Writing in the notes 'Jane has shown some improvement this term' is not good enough, as it is too subjective and will be meaningless to others reading it later on.

Change the programme in the light of progress – always be considering possible improvements in the programme and aim to provide an increasingly complex set of targets. Do not let your trainee remain on the same stage for long periods of time. Be aware that your trainee might *regress*. This may be because the steps are too large or the events being used to reinforce are no longer as effective. You must be prepared to change the programme if this happens.

Be consistent – a slow-learning individual learns best if those working with him are consistent in their approach. Use similar instructions; only change the tasks when the steps have been mastered; make sure your colleagues know how you are doing the teaching and which steps you have reached. It will be necessary to teach staff, parents and others involved so that everyone concerned uses an identical approach at all times.

CONCLUSION

The use of the principles of behaviour modification to teach the mentally handicapped is not easy. It will involve you in more methodical work, harder work and greater effort, *but* it will also offer a structured framework within which to work, objectives towards which to aim, and evidence of success with even the most handicapped of individuals. When previously helpless individuals learn how to feed and wash themselves, when they begin to communicate more appropriately and when they show increased social awareness of other people, then the effort becomes worthwhile.

In this short chapter, only the philosophy can be outlined and some practical guidance and examples given. The books listed in the bibliography are strongly recommended to readers who wish to become involved in programmes; the books should be consulted before any extensive behaviour modification programmes are begun.

Bibliography

Adaptive Behaviour Scale. (1974). (Washington, DC: American Association on Mental Deficiency)

Apex (The Journal of the British Institute of Mental Handicap) Kidderminster

Doll, E. A. (1963). *The Vineland Social Maturity Scale* (American Guidance Service Inc.)

Cunningham, C. C. and Jeffree, D. M., (1971). *Parental Involvement Project* (P.I.P.)

Ethical Implications of Behaviour· Modification (1977). Conference Proceedings. (British Institute of Mental Handicap, Kidderminster)

Fairview Self-Help Scale. (1970). (California: Fairview State Hospital)

Gardner, W. I. (1971). *Behaviour Modification in Mental Retardation.* (Chicago: Aldine, Atherton)

Gunzberg, H. C. (1974). *Progress Assessment Charts.* (Birmingham: SEFA Publications)

Haring, N. G. and Brown, L. J. (eds.) (1977). *Teaching the Severely Handicapped.* Vols I and II. (New York: Grune & Stratton)

Jackson, M. J. and Hattersley, J. (1974). *Teaching Self-Help Skills to the Mentally Handicapped using Behaviour Modification Techniques and Development of Play with Retarded Children.* (British Institute of Mental Handicap)

Jeffree, D. M. and McConkey, R. (1976). *PIP Developmental Charts.* (London: Hodder & Stoughton Educational)

Kiernan, C. C. (1974). Behaviour modification. In: Clarke, A. M. and Clarke, A. D. B. (eds.) *Mental Deficiency: the Changing Outlook.* (London: Methuen)

Kiernan, C. C. and Jones, M. (1978). *Behaviour Assessment Battery.* (Windsor: NFER)

Kiernan, C. C., Jordan, R. and Saunders, C. (1979). *Starting Off.* (London: Souvenir Press)

Mittler, P. (ed.) (1973). *Assessment for Learning in the Mentally Handicapped.* (London: Churchill Livingstone)

Perkins, E. A., Taylor, P. D. and Capie, A. C. M. (1976). *Helping the Retarded: A Systematic Behavioural Approach.* (Kidderminster: British Institute of Mental Handicap)

Schiefelbusch, R. L. (ed.) (1972). *The Language of the Mentally Retarded.* (Baltimore: University Park Press)

Skinner, B. F. (1974). *About Behaviourism.* (London: Jonathan Cape)

STAR: Social Training Achievement Record (1979). (Starcross: Royal Western Counties Hospital)

Thompson, T. and Grabowski, J. (1977). *Behaviour Modification of the Mentally Retarded.* 2nd Edn. (New York: Oxford University Press)

Williams, C. (1974). *Behaviour Modification for Nurses.* (Kidderminster: British Institute of Mental Handicap)

6

MENTAL ILLNESS IN THE MENTALLY HANDICAPPED

J. C. N. Tibbits

INTRODUCTION

The term *illness* implies that there has been a state of non-illness before the onset of discernible disorder, whereas the term *handicap* is used to express a disability of development which arises, and is most often recognizable, at an early age.

Nobody is immune either from handicap or illness. Some people are unusually vulnerable to them, either because of predispositions or damaging events in the body; because of psychological, social and spiritual stresses; or, most commonly, because of a combination of these very complex features of human nature and nurture.

INCIDENCE OF MENTAL ILLNESS IN MENTALLY HANDICAPPED PEOPLE

Mentally handicapped people are no less likely to incur super-added mental illness than other people are. There is evidence that those who come to the clinical attention of the mental handicap hospital may be *more* at risk. For example:

(a) In 1971, Primrose estimated that 60% of residents in mental handicap hospitals needed psychiatric treatment for the whole range of mental illnesses and problems, in addition to assistance in overcoming their more fundamental handicaps of mind.

(b) The 'major mental illnesses' were said to have occurred in the lives of some 14% of a sample of 300 mentally handicapped hospital residents; of these illnesses approximately half were schizophrenic psychoses, as compared with an incidence in the general population of from 1 to 2% (Tibbits, 1978).

These findings apply to that particular series of hospital residents only. No conclusions can be drawn about other hospitals, let alone the mentally handicapped people who are not hospitalized, or even under outpatient care.

In the past, a basic intellectual handicap may have obscured mental illness, the presentation of which, in the mentally handicapped, has been relatively little reported until recent times (Heaton-Ward, 1977).

Some of the literature, press reports, views of the public, and interpretations of the law relating to the mentally handicapped and the mentally ill confuse them. This suggests that they are similar conditions which pose problems and solutions of a similar kind. This is a serious distortion, and at the very least a misguided over-simplification of the human needs which are at stake.

Even today there remains a strong tendency to accept major disturbances of personality, mood and social behaviour in the mentally handicapped as though they were merely and auto-matically the natural outcome of that handicap, rather than to regard them as genuine pathological processes. Knowledge of the fundamental nature, causation and presentation of mental illness is itself far from satisfactory; this contributes to our inability to recognize it easily in a person who is mentally handicapped. The more severe the basic handicap the less easy, or even feasible, it is to diagnose a mental illness.

When a mentally handicapped person shows disturbances of personal state and behaviour patterns, these cannot be assumed to be just another set of problems arising from the basic handicap, especially when the upset is *out of character* with the individual's *previous personality*, and when it persists for more than a short while. The damaging consequences of inept care or the ignoring of mental signs and symptoms are no less serious than ineptitude in the handling of physical ailments.

NEUROSIS

This is the term used to describe the systematic manifestation of an abnormally high and persistent basal level of anxiety, perhaps accompanied by some degree of depression. This leads to a range of symptoms determined by the ways in which the individual deals with his raised, generalized anxiety. These ways are various, but none of them over-steps the bounds of what is reasonably intelligible to someone in a normal state of health. The neurotic condition does not severely impair such insight and ability to communicate as the individual has, either in degree or in kind, as does the psychosis.

Neuroses do not occur in a vacuum nor, necessarily, are they simply *internal* aspects of the individual concerned. The *context* is always important, and a detailed understanding and history-taking of past life and present situation, particularly in terms of relationships with others, is a vital part of accurate diagnosis.

A thorough initial physical check-up, with all the tests relevant to the symptoms, to exclude organic illness, and reassurance about physical complaints, usually lowers anxiety.

In the long-term neuroses, it is important to remember the possibility that a symptom or sign may arise due to some new physical disorder which is quite separate from the ongoing neurosis.

Types of Neurosis

It is helpful to consider neurotic states in terms of the following categories:

anxiety state
anxiety–depressive state
anxiety–hysteria
obsessive–compulsive state

It is rarely helpful to label a person as suffering from *hysteria*, as frequently hysterical signs and symptoms may, in the end, turn out to have been the superficial manifestation of a more serious underlying physical or psychological disturbance.

Symptoms and Signs of the Neuroses

Anxiety State

The various patterns of neurosis are maladaptive ways of dealing with rational and irrational problems in people whose temperament and personality include a high basic level of anxiety.

Anxiety is a reaction of the *whole person*. The physical features of fear are well known to all of us, and anxiety is a pattern of fear which most of us have experienced in some degree.

Anxiety can also be seen as excitement converted into a frustrated, and frustrating, fear; the person becomes, as it were, rooted to the spot of his or her dreads, and is unable to act appropriately whether by fight or flight. Much energy is diverted into vicious circles of self-preoccupation and tension of mind-and-body. The tensed musculature becomes a kind of armour, and is accompanied by an increase of the defences of the character-armour, so that 'neurotics' tend to demonstrate a rigidity of behaviour beyond the normal. The price to the individual, in order to maintain this pathological *status quo*, is high.

The patient may complain of his anxieties and tensions directly, or they may be presented less directly; as headaches or indigestion, for example.

In patients with little or no expressive language, as in many mentally handicapped people, one must rely on *observation* of their behaviour in order to understand that they are suffering from a neurosis, so that signs become more important than symptoms. Overt evidence of anxiety may be expressed in a direct form such as a visible tension, tremulousness, sweating, palpitations, loss of concentration, irritability, increasing fear of social situations, and perhaps phobic avoidance of particular experiences or contexts.

Anxiety – depression

This condition differs from the anxiety state in that an element of sadness and tearfulness and perhaps a more marked tendency to lack of sleep, in the form of *difficulty in getting off to sleep,* are present. The depressive element can be seen as another manifestation of the underlying anxiety, and is sometimes a reaction, and frequently an overreaction, to actual social circumstances.

Anxiety – hysteria

In this form, neurosis presents with the anxiety heavily masked by means of 'conversion' into untypical bodily complaints or into a range of manipulative behaviours.

Mixed Types of Anxiety – Neuroses

Many patients present a picture of illness which reflects a mixture of these three forms of anxiety-neurosis.

Example: Joe had always lived at home and attended ESN(S) school. His handicaps have made him very dependent on his mother, both practically and emotionally. He is very attached to his daily routine and becomes unhappy and frightened if it is upset. As he moved into adolescence the family's problem, and Joe's especially, was heightened by his difficulties in dealing with psychosexual development. Joe's anxiety was now constant; he was irritable, tremulous and easily cowed. He had bouts of weeping and also tantrums from time to time; his sleep was disturbed; and he showed signs of losing his rather precarious hold on self-help, communication and social skills. His mother became seriously ill, and Joe's anxiety-state became severe; it persisted even after her recovery. Treatment with Doxepin and Valium, together with consistent supportive reassurance for him, and regular family outpatient appointments, led to a general improvement. During this spell of intensive care it became clear that some of the patient's complaints of aches and pains were not straightforward bodily effects of anxiety, depression and tension, but were a further way of expressing his free-floating anxiety. These 'secondary' complaints had the manipulative quality of hysterical symptoms.

In this case-history, the features of all these types of anxiety-state are demonstrated.

69

Obsessive–Compulsive Neurosis

In an overanxious personality with marked guilt feelings, these attributes may become intensified and organized into obsessive ruminations and rituals of thought and behaviour to an irrational degree, as a full-blown neurosis. A common preoccupation is with sexual guilt feelings which become displaced onto ritual behaviours such as hand-washing.

Example: Herbert, a 24-year-old with Down's syndrome, spends many hours a day on washing and re-washing himself and his possessions. These ritual actions take complete precedence over the needs of ordinary living. If, by some means, these behaviours are prevented, massive anxiety and depression ensue.

Many handicapped people manifest a lesser degree of repetitive, stereotyped, obsessive–compulsive behaviour. Not all of them can be said to be suffering from true neurosis – some are underoccupied, some are suffering from one of the forms of autism, and some are manifesting a behaviour which is not fully intelligible in our present state of knowledge. The full-blown obsessive–compulsive disorder is difficult to treat because it occurs in very rigid, guilt-laden personalities.

Behaviour Disorders

Thus, we have seen that pathological anxiety may be dealt with inwardly, and in a suppressed self-punishing form, leading to tension of the mind-and-body; a neurosis. However, anxiety may provoke the individual to demonstrate his difficulties by *acting them out*, in terms of irritability, aggression, or other externalized antisocial symptoms.

Neurosis and Mental Handicap

It is sometimes said that the mentally handicapped do not incur prolonged neuroses, because they tend to release their anxieties in 'storms of affect' and hence accumulation of the problem into a syndrome or illness is said not to occur. This is not necessarily true; some mentally handicapped people are persistently overanxious, and will manifest obsessive rituals to keep the environment as stable and predictable as they can. They may show a degree of dependency on those who care for them well beyond that which may be attributed solely to their mental handicap.

There is evidence that neurosis involves a tendency to regress to the more primitive forms of behaviour of earlier life. In the mentally handicapped, whose maturity has been arrested at various levels of incompleteness, reversion to childlike behaviours easily occurs when anxiety is high. Regression, for example, in terms of self-help skills, finger-feeding, drinking only from a bottle on mother's knees, perhaps with a reversion to playing with faeces, or oral preoccupations, such as self-induced vomiting, can occur in adults, and may represent a sexualized version of infantile behaviour-patterns.

It is unprofessional to speak of psychiatric patients in terms of good–bad judgements. The important thing is to *understand* the processes which induce the behaviour and the internal upsets of the individual. This does not mean that handicapped people are immune from the consequences of their actions, in terms of responsibility; but it does mean that, if a clear diagnosis of neurosis or psychosis has been made, judgmental terms such as 'naughty' or 'mischievous' or 'always complaining' are best avoided, as they do not assist either in diagnosis or the appropriate treatment.

Management and Treatment of the Neuroses in the Mentally Handicapped

The basic concern is to diminish the level of anxiety by whatever means available, such as:

1. *Vector therapy.* A term covering efforts made to understand and, where possible, change the various social and psychological stresses on the individual in his current context, at home, in hospital or elsewhere.
2. *Relaxation therapy.* Where the handicapped patient is sufficiently accessible, relaxation therapy can be of help; this needs to be simply explained step by step, and regularly practised, under guidance. Basically, the principles are to reduce anxiety and tension, by way of reducing the physical

manifestations of muscle tension in limbs, trunk, head and neck.

3. *Personal attention and psychotherapy.* The neurotic sufferer should not be brushed aside as 'attention-seeking'. Merely to *accept* the need for attention is therapeutic. Regular opportunities for counselling conversations, which may need to be quite frequent at first and then gradually faded, are useful. Allowing over-attachment on a one-to-one basis is to be avoided. Behaviour-modification theory has shown us the danger of reinforcing and rewarding maladaptive behaviour. Personal psychotherapy is aimed, gently and with empathy, at reducing such behaviours, whilst accepting verbal (or even simple physical) expressions of them, strictly within the time and terms of the therapeutic interview.

4. *Medication.* There is a wide range of anxiety-reducing (anxiolytic) medications available. Some are discussed in Table 6.1.

Table 6.1 Some basic anxiolytic drugs

Approved name	Proprietary name	Approximate DAILY dose-range	Comments
Barbiturates	—	—	Commonly used in the past but there are now NO indications for the use of the barbiturates in treatment of mental illness.
Benzodiazepines Diazepam	Valium	10–50 mg	Diazepam is a reliable, safe anxiolytic. By intramuscular injection it is invaluable in calming patient, enabling vital investigations or treatments. Rare respiratory depression must be expected.
Propanediols Meprobamate	Equanil Miltown	400–2400 mg	A useful, muscle-relaxing anxiolytic.

The mentally handicapped have disorders of the central nervous system, and caution in the use of drugs acting on the central nervous system (CNS) is essential. Small initial doses, with gradual increase, are generally advisable.

Sometimes, small doses of antidepressive drugs, particularly those with an anxiolytic aspect, can be useful in the treatment of neurotic disorders. In the mentally handicapped, it is commonly found that the response is more rapid than in the non-handicapped. If there is no dramatic speedy response, it is wiser to persist for a reasonable time with one drug, rather than to juggle about with a series of different ones or combinations thereof.

The Treatment Context

Home or Hospital?

The onset of neurotic disorder, on top of the basic handicap, may be sufficient to severely disorganize a tenuous balance of domestic circumstances, where the patient is living in the family or in a small Home. At times it is necessary to admit the patient to hospital (as a day-patient or inpatient) for a period of stabilization. This should be considered *only* if pressure on the patient, and on those looking after him, have reached a serious pitch of crisis. A hospital is not always necessary for the treatment of neurosis, especially as behaviour and mental state may be quite different in different contexts and revert back to their former state on return to the original environment. It *is* always vital that the treatment team as a whole (family, physician, teachers, social workers, psychologists and others) should be working together for the same goals, in close co-ordination, and making the best use of whatever facilities are locally available for treatment.

Inevitably, the mentally handicapped person is considerably dependent upon others for his care. It is therefore important for everyone involved to know the living environment, whether home or elsewhere, and to understand the treatment; the side-effects, if any; the time involved and the outcome.

It is rare for a neurotic disorder *in itself* to call for compulsory admission to a hospital. Only if antisocial behaviour, for example serious sexual misconduct in public, has occurred, may this be considered necessary.

Eccentric sexual behaviours, and aggressive behaviours such as arson, may occur in some mentally handicapped people as a result of their immaturity and of the stresses under which they live. Such behaviour patterns, in the ordinary way, are likely to be manifestations of major mental disorder or of grave character-disorder if found in non-handicapped people; but they can often be seen as a sign of immaturity and perhaps learned behaviour in the mentally handicapped. One of the side-effects of in-stitutional treatment may be the acquisition of secondary sympt-toms and behaviours by mimicry of other residents.

We tend to expect handicapped people to be free of the social excesses which other members of society may display quite openly and seemingly without offence.

Outcome

The outcome of treatment varies according to the depth and duration of the neurotic disorder under treatment, but results are no more disappointing than in non-handicapped people; perseverance with treatment will usually result in some con-siderable amelioration, if not in complete relief.

It is necessary to stress again that an overall picture is essential, including full assessment of possible physical causation, or physical disorders concomitant with the neurosis. For example, people with mild temporal lobe abnormalities which do not produce identifiable epileptiform 'attacks' of any sort, can show a degree of irritability and explosiveness of behaviour which may be better controlled by an anticonvulsant such as Tegretol than by anxiolytics or antidepressives.

Electroplexy (ECT or electroconvulsive therapy) has no place in the treatment of neurotic disorders.

PSYCHOSIS

Differentiation from Neurosis

A psychosis, like a neurosis, is a serious change in the thoughts, feelings and behaviour of the sufferer: but *unlike* a neurosis, there is often no adequate discernible cause in terms of a reaction to personal stresses. Psychosis is also a more profound change than neurosis, and lies outside our everyday waking experience of self and others. A bizarre and alien quality helps us to distinguish a psychosis from a neurosis.

Types of Psychosis

It is useful to classify the psychoses as:

affective disorders
schizophrenic disorders
paranoid disorders
organic psychoses

The psychoses are generally regarded as *major* mental illnesses. The thoughts, feelings and behaviour of a psychotic person are likely to produce a state of diminished personal responsibility. There is little use, and may be real harm, in trying to convince a person suffering from psychosis that his or her irrational ideas and actions are unrealistic.

Often, very little interpersonal or behavioural therapy is possible, in the presence of severe psychosis, beyond strong and warm supportiveness and vigilance. At this stage, medication is the main treatment. That is not to say that medication is the whole answer, but it does enable the 'question' to become shareable, in most cases.

Signs and Symptoms of the Psychoses

Affective Psychoses

An affective psychosis is potentially a bipolar illness, in that the patient's whole functioning, and especially the affect (the overall mood) is either abnormally lowered (depressed) at the one pole, or abnormally elevated (hypomanic or manic) at the other. Depressive illness is more frequent in the mentally handicapped than its hypomanic or manic counterpart. Both are severe and often apparently self-generating illnesses.

Depression in this context bears only slight resemblances to what most people experience of *everyday* mood swings. Perhaps someone who has been through a severe bereavement crisis, and through the first 18 months of gradual adjustment, may have some real notion of the quality and the degree of a psychotic depressive illness.

Signs and Symptoms of Depression

Some of the manifestations of depressive psychosis are open to observation, from without, as clinical *signs*; it may even be possible to make a firm diagnosis when the basic handicaps make it extremely difficult or impossible to obtain any subjective data, i.e. symptoms, from the patient:

1. Everything loses its appeal and tends to become positively unpleasant, fearsome and dark.
2. All functions are impaired, from rational assessment of self and others, through to bowel functioning.
3. The impairment consists both of slowing, and of distortion by feelings of guilt and unworthiness.
4. This 'guilt' may be experienced directly as such, or in terms of some bodily fear such as of a malignant growth of the bowel.
5. Loss of sleep is often severe, and characteristically *early and despair-loaded awakening* in the small hours occurs (whereas, in the 'depressive reaction' of the neurotic type, it is more commonly a difficulty in getting off to sleep).
6. Loss of concentration, hope and self-esteem in varying degrees,
   loss of all drive and libido;
   loss of appetite for food;
   loss of ability to cry is a frequent concomitant of loss of ability to laugh.
7. Guilt feelings may become so strong and bizarre that they are truly delusional in quality. (A delusion is an idea or system of ideas which is both unrelated to objective reality and also not accessible to reasoning or correction by discussion.)
8. Delusions may be projected outwards, and so acquire a secondary paranoid nature. For example, a middle-aged hospital resident, Mrs M., believed that she was being 'booked'

by the staff for offences, which were in fact offences only against the patient's own internal depressed and obsessive standards.

9. Particularly in middle age and later life, psychotic depression often brings about an exaggeration of an over-scrupulous, obsessional personality, during the episode.

10. General slowing of function is usual, and yet there may also, at the same time, be a *thought-race* happening, with obsessive rumination on past sorrows and 'sins'.

11. There is often visible and aimless agitation. Hand-wringing and repetition of sad phrases may be observed.

12. The facies is a mask of down-turned sorrow.

13. A frequent accompaniment of the early-waking pattern is the so-called *diurnal variation*; the patient feels and appears much less disturbed and ill as the day wears on, and it is therefore vital in assessment to see the person in the morning, when things are at their worst.

14. *Suicide is a real risk*, and is increased:

    (a) As a very slowed-up person begins to improve, and then may find the drive to act on the fixed idea that his family, friends, and he himself will be better off with him dead, for example. This is a very different situation from the depression of neurosis, wherein suicide hints or gestures are not infrequent, but are aimed at trying to relieve a life situation rather than to end life.

    (b) With the evidently depressed person who smiles over the top of his depression, however unconvincingly; the so-called 'smiling-depression'.

    (c) In the early hours of the day.

    (d) In life situations where the patient is exposed to many (perhaps conflicting) pressures.

    (e) When ideas of guilt and incurability are heightened by the ill-judged, all too frequent advice of others, e.g. 'pull yourself together'.

    (f) When an actual loss occurs (e.g. of a supportive person) or a felt loss becomes intensified.

Management and Treatment of Depressive Psychosis

Management

During a depressive episode the patient will certainly need great support, particularly during the profound phase. The depression may very well make him appear unable to believe that any change for the better is possible, but firm reassurance, together with a genuine personal belief in one's appropriate methods of therapy, may well see a suicidal patient through an otherwise irreversible illness. Medication is necessary once thorough care-team assessment, including full physical examination, has been made. The intensity of this medication, and of general care, depend on the severity of the illness, and the first decision to be made is where to treat the patient.

At Home – If the depression is mild, and if there is a reasonably supportive environment – particularly if community intensive nursing support is available, coupled with reasonable co-operation from the patient and family – it is desirable to avoid hospitalization, even as a day-patient, but frequent reviews and cautious use of medication are essential.

In Hospital – The advantages of complete or partial hospitalization include more intensive opportunities for interaction with skilled staff, and prevention of secondary symptoms due to isolation, under-occupation,˙ and prolonged rumination without support. There is no 'magic' about a hospital or day-centre. The decision depends to some extent on the quality of facilities available in such a unit.

If there is clear evidence of major depressive illness with strong suicidal drives, there should be no hesitation in advising hospitalization as an inpatient, for a short period at least, during the crisis and until improvement has been consolidated.

The vexed question of compulsory admission – in the case of the patient where two competent doctors are satisfied that suicide is a major risk (or that prolonged damage to useful social function is probable) – then it may seem wise for social worker or relative to apply for a short-term admission order. This whole question of informal or compulsory admission is debatable in each case, but must be kept in mind in most cases. Whatever course is followed must be entirely in the interest of, and for the benefit of, the patient.

ECT (Electroplexy/Electroconvulsive Therapy)

Another matter of serious debate is the increasingly disfavoured ECT. It may be thought that there still are patients for whom ECT is a life-saver. It should never be given without consent of the patient and/or the guardian, and never without full consultant–anaesthetist induction and after-care. These comments apply to its use in *any* of the psychiatric syndromes, of which depressive psychosis is the most likely to respond to appropriate use of ECT. Premature use of ECT makes for a false alleviation or suppression of symptoms, and hence may actually render relapse more likely. Repeated courses of ECT are known to have caused some degree of permanent brain-damage, which is quite different from the short-term memory impairment caused by a particular course of the treatment, which will usually lift in a few weeks.

Drug Therapy

In most cases the medication of choice is probably a tricyclic antidepressant drug. These drugs generally do not begin to produce clinical change for 1–2 weeks. Some people find the side-effects most distressing, but these usually lift in a few days. If they persist, a change of drug will be required.

It seems wise to become fully competent and at home with the dosages and effects of one or two antidepressives in the treatment of depressive illness in mentally handicapped people, and to adhere to their usage as a basic practice. Doxepin, like amitripyline, has a useful added anxiolytic effect. Either of these drugs may, at times, be given once daily at night to aid sleep and so that side-effects are less troublesome to the patient. Dothiapin is a useful drug, with fewer side-effects and lower risk of triggering epileptic attacks.

These three drugs (doxepin, dothiapin and amitriptyline) seem to achieve satisfactory therapeutic effect in doses of up to 75 mg daily. Allowance must of course be made for the patient's age, tolerance, body-weight and general condition; and the dosage calculated with caution – if necessary building the dose up gradually, unless the severity of the depression demands very pressing action.

Outcome

There is usually a satisfactory outcome within a few weeks, but continued support and surveillance is necessary, as depressive disorders show a tendency to recurrence. Also many handicapped people who undergo depression have a fragile basic personality, and may be the more easily triggered into relapses.

Table 6.2 Some basic antidepressive drugs

Approved name	Proprietary name	Approximate DAILY dose-range (mg)	Comments: indications and side-effects
Tricyclics			All tend to produce similar basic side-effects: 1. Commonest are excessive sweating, postural hypotension, visual-accommodation problems, dry mouth, constipation; sometimes urinary retention 2. More dangerous: cardio-vascular effects (said to be least with doxepin but are reported with amitriptyline). These effects extend from abnormal ECG through to cardiac dis-rhythmias and even, very rarely, fatal ventricular fibrillation; in the elderly, congestive cardiac failure 3. These drugs are to varying extents liable to trigger epileptic attacks. Use with maximum caution in patients with glaucoma (a serious eye condition), prostatism (enlargement of the prostate gland), heart disease and epilepsy
Doxepin	Sinequan	25–150	An effective antidepressive

80

Table 6.2 (*cont.*)

Approved name	Proprietary name	Approximate DAILY dose-range (mg)	Comments: indications and side-effects
			drug with marked anxiolytic effect. Low risk, if any, of cardiovascular toxicity
Dothiapin	Prothiaden	25–150	Said to act more quickly than amitriptyline; fewer side-effects; less likely to trigger epilepsy
Amitriptyline	Tryptizol	10–150	Some anxiolytic effects. Risk of triggering epileptic attacks. Cardiovascular toxicity must be cautiously considered
Monoamine oxidase inhibitors (MAOIs)			These not as safe or as useful antidepressants as tricyclics: 1. Occasionally produce severe acute hypertension, especially with foodstuffs containing significant amounts of tyramine, e.g. cheeses, some wines, yeast products, animal livers, bananas, and broad bean pods 2. May enhance effects of amines which are contained in many easily obtained medicines for upper respiratory tract infections (i.e. of the nose, throat, larynx and chest) 3. Prolong and potentiate the central effects of pethidine and other narcotic drugs 4. Can interact with *anti*-hypertensive drugs to produce severe *hypertensive crises* 5. Dangerous to give these drugs with tricyclic drugs because of unpredictable potentiation effects
Tranylcypromine	Parnate	10–30	May cause liver damage

Note: In addition, one of the benzodiazepine drugs, as Diazepam, may be very helpful in relieving anxiety and agitation during the day.

81

Symptoms and Signs of Hypomania and Mania

In about half of the 14% of the hospitalized mentally handicapped patients examined by the author (Tibbits, 1978) who suffer from psychotic illness, this is of the affective type: 3% depressive and just over 1% manic or hypomanic. Hypomania and mania are thus the less frequent affective disorders in the mentally handicapped. Hypomania, which is more common than full, developed mania, is manifested in hyperactivity with restlessness and sleeplessness, even to the point of exhaustion, together with grandiose ideas and a kind of angry jocundity. In full mania, the anger may become frank aggression, the hyperactivity become overwhelmingly incessant night and day, and there is a real danger of inanition and exhaustion resulting.

Particularly in the mentally handicapped, the differential diagnosis between mania, states of high excitement in schizophrenics, and extreme episodes in normally hyperactive people can be difficult. Characteristically, the manic patient shows flights of ideas and incessant chatter of speech with very shallow, laughable associations. It is a serious error to laugh *at* (or even *with*) hypomanic and manic patients, since those who have recall after the illness often bitterly resent you for having laughed *against* them. One view of the manic syndrome is that it is a flight from an underlying depression, and, whether this is true or not, it will do no harm to remember that, whatever appearances may suggest, the patient is *not* happy or amused at his state, or the reaction of others towards it.

Mixed Affective Disorder (Manic-Depression)

Example: Elsie is aged 45 years and has for some years shown repeated spells when she is unable to cope with her share of household chores. She becomes very slow and sad, and loses all her interests and vitality. She eats and sleeps little during these spells. She wakes at about 3 a.m. and is very distressed and tearful until early afternoon. Once, she became hypomanic and was restless, excited and noisy; she seemed over-cheerful, but there were episodes of explosive irritability.

Management and Treatment of Hypomania and Mania

The acute phase may be effectively brought under control with thioridazine (Melleril), chlorpromazine, or a butyrophenone such as haloperidol. There may be a need to give these drugs intramuscularly, until the patient is calm enough to take oral medication. With haloperidol (Serenace) it is advisable to give an anti-parkinsonian drug, for example, procyclidine (Kemadrin) in a daily dose-range of 2.5–30 mg. Quite large doses of neuroleptic drugs (i.e. major tranquillizers), in divided doses, are likely to be required for a while; then, medication in maintenance doses should be continued for weeks or months after control has been restored.

Lithium carbonate, which is available as the standard tablet (Camcolit) or as the longer-acting Priadel, may be felt to be a useful aid in control and prophylaxis of recurrent and treatment-resisting manic and hypomanic disorders. It is vital to monitor the dosage given very carefully by means of frequent plasma-level estimations, to keep the level below 1.2 mmol/l. Above that level, toxic effects appear and above 1.6 mmol/l, the toxicity becomes really very dangerous. A safe and usually effective range of lithium plasma-level is between 0.6 mmol/l and 1.2 mmol/l. Twice-weekly monitoring is the *absolutely minimal* safe standard practice during the first few weeks of treatment; gradually reducing to fortnightly or monthly estimations.

Early signs of toxicity are general malaise, fine tremor of the hands, nausea and abdominal discomfort. Later, drowsiness with vomiting and diarrhoea indicate dangerously rising toxicity; the drug must be stopped immediately, and urgent serial blood levels be obtained. Severe lithium poisoning causes coma and death; haemodialysis (a complex technique for blood filtration which requires specialized intensive care in a general hospital) may be required to avert this. Lithium is contraindicated in patients with a history of renal or cardiac disease, and should be offered only with the greatest circumspection to a patient with hypothyroidism, since lithium may lead to overt myxoedema. A probable safe and therapeutic dose-range of lithium is 0.5–1.5 g/day.

Hospitalization is required during the initial treatment and stabilization of lithium dosage.

In the management of these states it is important to have intramuscular tranquillizing agents available, since the state may fluctuate quite wildly, and urgent control be required. In the extremely disturbed patient it will be necessary to keep a careful monitoring of fluid and dietary intake, and to take all steps to avoid collapse from exhaustion. Staff must be prepared for possible violence, even in apparently jokey and previously non-violent persons.

Outcome

Most hypomanic and manic episodes can be brought under control within weeks, but relapse is a serious possibility and long-term supportive surveillance may well be required, with the discreet use of maintenance medication.

The Schizophrenic Psychoses

Symptoms and Signs

Classically, schizophrenia is broken down, in terms of the type of symptoms and signs displayed, into the simple, hebephrenic, paranoid, and rare catatonic types. In the mentally handicapped, it can be difficult to discern the insidious changes of the simple type, but there is much less reason for failure of early diagnosis in the other types.

A schizophrenic is someone who is experiencing and manifesting a profound fragmentation of personality, with thought disorder, affective dislocation, and spells of intense terror, especially when hallucinations or delusions are pressing hard. Hallucinations are auditory, visual or bodily experiences and sensations which are not brought about by the environment.

The illness may show an acute fulminating, or insidious, onset. The basic mental change seems to be an inexplicable sense that the self and the world are different from their former state, and that the boundaries of self and others are disturbingly distorted. Things and people may seem to be invading and influencing the mind in novel and disturbing ways. Thoughts appear as though alien to the self, and they influence conduct in bizarre fashions. Although outwardly withdrawn and sluggish, a patient may experience racing and disconnected thoughts. Classically, the schizophrenic patient shows the following patterns:

1. Emotionally cut off, and likely to show a mood-tone which is monotonous and not related to the current situation (flat and incongruous affect). There may be, however, evident high anxiety, depression or elation; these states may be succeeded one by another in a bewildering chaos.

2. A chilly aloofness (hauteur) often predominates, particularly when the paranoid syndrome is marked.

3. Even when the patient is facetious and punning, the examiner rarely feels like making a happy response, unlike the situation in the manic states.

4. Associations between spoken thoughts or behaviours may be indecipherable, and impulsiveness may be expected, sometimes even in an apparently stuporose patient.

5. Any clouding of consciousness makes the diagnosis of schizophrenia suspect, and investigations for organic causes, including temporal lobe abnormalities, are indicated.

6. Persecutory ideas (paranoid delusions) are often accounted for as the patient's effort to come to terms with the bizarre changes in his personal experience of self and others.

7. Hallucinatory voices may give commands, and the response of the patient may be violence to himself or others. The patient may visibly listen to the voices and/or converse with them.

8. The capacity of willed activity (volition) is seriously impaired, and inability to reach decisions or to act upon them is typical.

9. Some patients feel that they are totally operated from outside themselves.

10. Catatonia may take the form of intense excitement with frantic purposeless activity, or it may appear as a stuporose state in which strange, statuesque postures may be adopted and maintained; on examination, the famous 'waxy flexibility' of limbs may be demonstrated, when the limbs will be held by the patient in whatever position the examiner places them. This seems to be part of a pattern of automatic obedience, but on the other hand there may be total negativism, or alternating states of negativism and automatism.

Example: Mary is only moderately handicapped, and her mother brought her to the outpatient clinic at age 23 because she had noticed such a change in her daughter's personality. Previously fairly outgoing and sociable, Mary had, over a few weeks, become solitary and withdrawn.

She muttered to herself and appeared to be experiencing voices unheard by other people. She would giggle for no good reason on occasion, and sometimes this seemed to be socially quite inappropriate behaviour. Her mother noticed a' loss of warmth in Mary's relationship with her and others. At interview, Mary managed to convey that voices did come to her, and sometimes told her to do 'naughty things'. She had lost all concern for her previous interests. Her mood was not depressed or elevated, but flattened and indifferent. She said 'they have changed me' and 'it is the telly, it speaks to me'.

Management and Treatment of Schizophrenia (see Table 6.3)

Both management and treatment will depend on the current state and history of the particular patient, but at all times delicacy and caution are required. Medication is usually mandatory, particularly in the control of the acute state. Generally maintenance medication is necessary over months or years. It is important to achieve a balance; neither stultifying the patient with excessive doses on the one hand, nor leaving him vulnerable to explosive impulsiveness and misery on the other hand.

Treatment Context

Management and treatment at home. This is frequently possible, except in very acute schizophrenic states, particularly with the use of ongoing medication, competent community nursing, and frequent medical attention.

Hospital treatment. Whether as a day- or inpatient, it may well be necessary to admit to hospital in order to achieve a sufficient degree of stabilization in order safely to return the patient home. Duration of stay in hospital should be as short as safely possible, and legal compulsion should only be used when known risk of

Table 6.3 Some basic drugs for use in treatment of schizophrenia and paranoid states

Approved name	Proprietary name	Approximate DAILY dose-range	Comments
Phenothiazines			Tardive CNS disorders may arise after prolonged administration
Chlorpromazine	Largactil	Acutely disturbed patient: 300–900 mg; otherwise: 50–300 mg	The standard drug of this class: irritability and/or drowsiness, depression, hypotension, cholestatic jaundice, sun-sensitivity, rare blood dyscrasias, epileptogenesis, and extra-pyramidal disorders occur: An anti-parkinsonian drug may be required to prevent the latter
Thioridazine	Melleril	50–300 mg	Syrup is useful. Lower toxicity and side-effects than Largactil: perhaps not as potent
Trifluoperazine	Stelazine	2–15 mg	May stimulate inert patients, but risk of provoking restlessness
Fluphenazine decanoate	Modecate	Test dose (intramuscular) 12.5 mg, then 25 mg every 2–4 weeks	Depot preparation. Extrapyramidal effects may be severe: use with an anti-parkinsonian drug (such as Kemadrin) *essential*. May precipitate depression
Phenylbutylperidines Pimozide	Orap	2–10 mg as a single daily dose	May equal effectiveness of Modecate, but oral. Use with an anti-parkinsonian drug such as Kemadrin essential (Falloon, Watt and Shepherd, 1978)
Butyrophenones Haloperidol	Serenace	1–10 mg	Useful drug, controls hyperactivity: but strong extra-pyramidal CNS effects. Use with an anti-parkinsonian drug such as Kemadrin essential
Benperidol	Anquil	0.25–1.5 mg	Not a very powerful anti-psychotic, but helps some problems of antisocial sexuality. Use with an anti-parkinsonian drug may be required

violence to self or others, or acute distress of patient and/or family, dictates this.

There is no mental illness in which accuracy of case-taking and study of family dynamics can be more helpful. Although the primary process of the psychosis may not be related to social circumstances and relationship structures, the outcome and everyday management is certainly profoundly affected by such insights.

Outcome

There are instances of complete recovery from short, strong schizophrenic episodes; but, in the main, this condition is only subject to control and requires long-term medication and ongoing support of the patient and those caring for him. Long-acting intramuscular drugs may help to avoid the relapses due to failure to take medication steadily. Some relapses may be of a mainly affective type, or present a mixed schizophrenic-affective picture.

Paranoid Psychoses

Symptoms and Signs

Paranoid disorders can occur without a background of affective or schizophrenic illness. The degree may vary from mild intermittent spells of heightened anxiety and grousing, right through to a florid state of incessant persecutory delusions and hallucinations. It has been demonstrated recently (Manschrak and Petri, 1978) that such paranoid states may occur in the very wide range of neurological disorders, sex chromosome disorders, metabolic illnesses, endocrine disorders, infectious diseases, abuse of alcohol and other social drugs, and various psychosocial conditions in the elderly.

Paranoid states may, therefore, be presenting features of a number of conditions; this serves to re-stress the need for the most thorough all-round assessment of every patient, both physically and mentally.

Treatment of Paranoid Psychoses (see Table 6.3)

Organic Psychoses

Mental handicaps are themselves organic impairments of intellectual and other mental functions – the so-called ('Amentias'; so the diagnosis of dementia is not always obvious or easy, since it consists of the symptoms and signs of irreversible deterioration of intellectual and other mental functions from a previously higher level. Mental handicap gives no immunity from any other organic mental impairment, however much it may tend to cloud the diagnosis.

Senile Dementia

Example: Kate was handicapped (Down's syndrome) and aged 50 years. Her family noticed a general deterioration in her memory, social abilities and energies. The diagnoses of depression or intercurrent illness having been gradually excluded, it became clear that the patient was ageing rapidly and suffering from a senile dementia. The age of onset is much earlier than in a normal adult, in line with the foreshortened life-span due to her basic handicap. It may be that arteriosclerosis is a factor in her dementia.

Pre-senile Dementia (Alzheimer's and Pick's diseases)

The picture is very similar to that of senile dementia but occurs in middle age.

Confusional States

These are characterized by clouding of consciousness, memory disorders, disorientation and often perceptual disorders (e.g. tactile hallucinations) and restlessness (as in the classic 'delirium').

Diagnosis and relief of the underlying cause will restore mental function, although, if the condition has been severe and prolonged, there may be residual dementia. Severe infections, intoxications, head injuries, dehydration, uraemia, myxoedema, cerebral hypoxia (commonly owing to cardiorespiratory deficiency) and drug or alcohol abuse are some not uncommon causes.

Secondary Dementias

Among the causes of progressive secondary dementia are long-standing alcohol abuse, brain injury, intracranial space-occupying lesions, malignant deposits, chronic cerebral hypoxia, tertiary syphilis and severe and intractable epilepsy.

It may be difficult to be sure, in a newly met patient, how much of the deficit is due to inherent handicap and how much due to dementing change. Careful history-taking and psychological testing are essential. Recent memory is lost in dementia more rapidly and severely than remote memory.

FEATURES IN MENTAL HANDICAP (see Table 6.4)

The whole process of diagnosis is made more difficult by basic communication problems; therefore it is essential to listen carefully to those who already know the patient well, and also to allow much time for the assessment.

Aids to Eliciting Accurate Information

1. It is necessary to *shape* questions so as to help the patient or informant, but it is also necessary to avoid so wording questions as to shape the answers in advance; particularly if the ground to be covered is subtle or unfamiliar to the person questioned.
2. Being questioned (interrogations), may cause real panic and 'false admissions' are a likely result. This risk is increased by the use of language which is too sophisticated for the patient or informant.
3. Panic may amount to the reaction of 'catastrophic anxiety' and block any ability to answer, or even lead to fight-or-flight behaviour.
4. Questions which extract facts, but ignore their context in the present and/or their roots in past history, will yield distorted evidence.
5. By their very nature questions demand answers; such a demand may be resented (even when reasonable, from the

Table 6.4 Some features which help to differentiate mental illnesses

Neuroses	Psychoses
(A) *Contact with the Patient*	
1. Possible with a patient who is basically approachable and able to hold a reasonable conversation	1. Schizophrenia: the patient is 'in a world of his own' and 'behind a wall of glass' Paranoid states: the patient's delusions dominate his life and he is cut off by them Organic psychoses: loss of recent memory, clouding of consciousness and disorientation make rational conversation difficult
(B) *Thought Contents*	
2. No evidence of thought disorder, delusions or hallucinations	2. Clear evidence of thought disorder, and of delusions and hallucinations, usually available
(C) *Response of the Patient*	
3. However disabled by the illness, the patient's responses usually seem appropriate to the interviewer	3. Responses are mostly inappropriate and often inexplicable because of the processes listed at 1 and 2 above

interviewer's viewpoint) and lead to emotionally distorted responses.

6. The preconceptions of all concerned (examiner, patient and informants) are always at work: it is necessary to 'read between the lines' and pick up the less obvious messages; e.g. the feeling-tone of the interview, the non-verbal communications which occur (gestures, expressions, silences, etc.); also comments which are voiced between more formal statements.

CONCLUDING REMARKS ABOUT CAUSATION, TREATMENT AND CARE OF MENTAL ILLNESS IN HANDICAPPED PEOPLE

Attention Giving

Whilst compassion and empathy are never misplaced, over-involvement emotionally in a particular attachment to a patient is unprofessional and promotes neurotic dependency.

91

Attention Seeking

There is nothing wrong with seeking attention, it is one of the necessities of the sick and handicapped. However, to foster and encourage attention-seeking behaviour can be a collusion with the very illness which one is allegedly trying to cure. On the whole, methods which strengthen the patient's identity and are *rewarding* to him do work, whereas methods which condescend to the patient, and are *punishing* to him, do not work. The matter is complicated, since apparent punishment may be gratifying to the patient. Therapists are not qualified to *judge*, but must assess.

Collusion with Sick Dependency

Whilst change may be secretly yearned after, human groups persistently cling to what is familiar and expect group members to comply with fixed roles. This also happens *within* individuals; for example, in the case of people who find abandonment of their invalidism extremely difficult. The living conditions of many mentally handicapped people reinforce a low level of self-esteem, a fragile self-image, and a poor grasp of the real existence and needs of other people (Wylie and Thomas, 1978). They often show anxious subservience, perhaps with counter-reactions in the form of aggressiveness. They tend to hold themselves stiffly (muscle-armour) and their personalities may appear rigid and stereotyped (character-armour). In their emotional and practical dependence on mothers or other caretakers, the handicapped may be held back from their best chance of solving the key problems of developing more self-confidence and maturity. It is not difficult for parents and care-staff to go along unwittingly colluding with this dependency, beyond what is absolutely required by the actual core handicap. Such collusion, however well meaning and/or unrealized, fosters immaturity and so fosters the increased likelihood of mental illness sooner or later.

References

Primrose, D. A. (1971). A survey of 502 consecutive admissions to a subnormality hospital from 1st January 1968 to 31st December 1970. *Br. J. Ment Subnorm., Subnorm.*, 27, 25

Heaton-Ward, A. (1977). Psychosis in mental handicap. *Br. J. Psychiatry.*, **130**, 525

Tibbits, J. C. N. (1978). A joint approach to domiciliary support. *Apex*, **6, 6**
Apex, **6, 26**

Wylie, B. and Thomas, C. (1978). Social skills training – a follow-up study. *Apex*, **6, 2**

Falloon, I., Watt, D. C. and Shepherd, M. (1978). A comparative trial of pimozide and fluphenazine decanoate in the continuation therapy of schizophrenia. *Psychol. Med.*, **8,** 59

Manschrak, T. C. and Petri, M. (1978). The paranoid syndrome. *Lancet*, **ii, 251**

Suggestions for Further Reading

Searles, H. F. (1965). *Collected Papers on Schizophrenia and Allied Subjects,* exp. chap. 24. (London: Hogarth Press and Institute of Psychoanalysis)

Crowcroft, A. (1967). *The Psychotic.* (Harmondsworth: Pelican original)

Silverstone, T. and Turner, P. (1974). *Drug Treatment in Psychiatry.* (London: Routledge & Kegan Paul Ltd)

Oswin, M. (1978). *Holes in the Welfare Net.* (London: Bedford Square Press and the NCSS)

Biestek, F.P., s.j. (1961). *The Casework Relationship.* (London: George Allen & Unwin)

Anderson, E. W. and Trethowan, W. H. (1973). *Psychiatry.* (London: Baillière Tindall)

7

EPILEPSY

B. I. Sacks

Management of the severely retarded tends to be characterized by the twin problems of maladaptive behaviour and chronic medical disorder. Of the latter one of the commonest is epilepsy. Approximately one-quarter of the severely subnormal have epileptic disorders and it is, therefore, important that those who are involved in the care of the handicapped are familiar with the diagnosis and management of this condition.

Although epilepsy is compatible with a wide range of intellectual ability it seems clear that the incidence of epilepsy rises relentlessly as the degree of handicap increases.

The frequency of epilepsy in the mildly mentally handicapped is very much less than in the severely subnormal, supporting the view that epilepsy in the latter group is mainly due to coarse brain damage.

This has obvious implications concerning management and prognosis and accounts for the well-known difficulties encountered in this group of patients.

RELATIONSHIP BETWEEN SEIZURES, DISTURBED BEHAVIOUR AND MENTAL RETARDATION

It is extremely difficult to unravel the relationships between disturbed behaviour, mental handicap and fits since there are so many variables involved. However, it has been shown that the presence of fits is associated with a higher percentage of disturbed behaviour and similarly difficult behaviour is commoner in the mentally handicapped.

In a study of disturbed behaviour in three hospitals, Eyman *et al.* (1969) showed that aggressive behaviour, attacks on other patients, hyperactivity, co-ordination difficulties and speech problems were more common in mentally handicapped patients with seizures than without seizures.

This association, however, was not shown in the Camberwell study. These studies are not comparable (only a quarter of the patients in the Camberwell study were institutionalized) but it may be that, although the presence of epilepsy does contribute to behaviour disorder, other factors such as a favourable family environment may be more important.

CAUSE OF EPILEPSY

From the point of view of causation, epilepsy is generally divided into two main groups: idiopathic (or epilepsy of unknown cause) and epilepsy with known causation.

The causes of epilepsy are legion and a specialized text should be consulted for an account of these. In the field of mental handicap known causes are much more commonly associated with epilepsy since both epilepsy and mental handicap may be caused by brain disorders of almost any kind. It is, therefore, of particular importance that all patients with fits be extensively investigated in an attempt to discover a cause for the seizures, since the cause may be treatable and may also have genetic and prognostic implications. Unfortunately the number of treatable conditions is disappointingly small.

Fits presenting for the first time in later life need adequate and rapid investigation since they may be due to abscesses or tumours of the brain.

In the severely handicapped the situation may be complicated by the fact that their threshold for fits is lower than normal, and seizures may be precipitated by infections. These fits cease spontaneously once the temperature is back to normal.

Whether the cause is due to recognizable underlying pathology or is unknown the epilepsy should be treated with the same energy and optimism, since fits resulting from severe brain damage may be modified or even sometimes suppressed for lengthy periods with modern methods of management.

THE DIAGNOSIS OF EPILEPSY

The diagnosis of epilepsy rests almost entirely on the history, and since there is no memory for the seizure an accurate description of events from reliable witnesses is essential. It is important to obtain an objective description of the event, and the distinction between the clinical description of the behaviour and the personal opinion of the observer must be emphasized. A great deal of information may be obtained by asking the witness to demonstrate the fit. Shyness on the part of observers may sometimes be overcome by a demonstration by the enquirer. In addition the following items should always be investigated:

date of first attack;
apparent precipitating events such as fever, trauma, onset of illness;
time of second and subsequent attacks, interval between attacks, especially in females, and whether they occur in bouts;
whether attacks occur at any special time of day or night;
change in frequency of attacks;
whether patient was cyanosed or not and the extent of this;
whether there were warnings of any kind;
the nature of onset of the attack – local or general, gradual or sudden;
whether consciousness was lost or not;
whether clonic tonic or other movements were shown, and what type and which muscle groups were affected;
if injuries were sustained;
if incontinence of urine, faeces or both, occurred;
the duration of the fit;
condition after the fit – whether sleepy, whether there was paralysis of any kind, automatic movements, or mental disturbance;

what treatment is being used, and the effect of treatment; whether several attacks occurred sequentially without the subject regaining consciousness in between.

The routine assessment of suspected epileptics should also include electroencephalography (EEG).

In most cases the diagnosis will become clear if information can be obtained on the above factors, particularly if the attack is typical of one of the main types in the classification. However, there are many conditions with which epilepsy can be confused (see Differential Diagnosis).

It is just as important to exclude the diagnosis of epilepsy as it is to make it. The implications of an incorrect diagnosis are serious since this would almost always involve prolonged drug treatment as well as inappropriate management and stress and anxiety in the patient's family.

CLASSIFICATION

It has proved difficult to obtain agreement on an international classification of epilepsy. The following is modified from the classification of the International League Against Epilepsy.

The modern classification of epilepsy is divided into two main groups – generalized and focal.

The two important groups under the first heading are *tonic clonic massive* or *grand mal* and *absences* or *petit mal*.

The most important type under the second heading is *complex partial* or *temporal lobe epilepsy.*

I. GENERALIZED
These are bilaterally symmetrical fits without focal onset.
(A)   Primary
     (i)   Tonic clonic massive (grand mal)
     (ii)   Absences (petit mal) infantile spasms
     (iii)   Massive myoclonic
                      myoclonic spasms
(B)   Secondary
     (i)   Tonic clonic (cause known)

II. PARTIAL or FOCAL
(A)   With elementary symptomatology (focal; Jacksonian; adversive)
(B)   With complex symptomatology: complex partial (temporal lobe; psychomotor)
(C)   Partial seizures with secondary generalization.

III. UNILATERAL

IV. UNCLASSIFIED
The term 'pyknolepsy', in which the patient may have hundreds of attacks of petit mal in a day, is no longer used.

THE CLINICAL PICTURE

It is generally felt that epilepsy *per se* does not produce mental changes unless the fits are severe enough to produce brain damage due to lack of oxygen.

Grand Mal

Pre-Ictal Symptoms

These may precede the seizure by hours or even days. They include irritability, depression, insomnia, vivid dreams, difficult and/or aggressive behaviour, giddiness and sudden twitches. Such symptoms may reach a crescendo immediately preceding an attack, after which the patient may feel better.

Precipitating Factors

These are usually difficult to identify but possibly include infections (in epileptics on medication), constipation, and many physical disorders.

In reflex epilepsy flickering lights may precipitate an attack. Some children move their fingers between their eyes and a light source to induce an attack.

The Aura

It is not usually possible to obtain a record of this in mentally handicapped persons, although it occurs in a majority of cases. It is produced by the beginning of the epileptic discharge and perceived before consciousness is lost; its form depends upon the focus of origin of the fit.

The aura may consist of the following: feelings of unreality (*jamais vu*), familiarity (*deja vu*), or fear. This may cause the patient to run without apparent reason and then fall unconscious. There may be hallucinations of any type, vertigo, sensations of many kinds including pain and motor auras which may involve any muscle group, sometimes with organized movements such as smacking the lips.

The convulsion may begin with a *cry* which is harsh in quality and is due to the forcible expiration of air through the partly closed vocal cords.

Consciousness is lost and the patient falls to the ground and may injure himself. Scars and bruises are common in epileptics for this reason.

The phase of *tonic spasm* (continuous tension or contraction of muscles) is now obvious with symmetrical adduction of arms which are flexed at the elbows and wrists, while the legs are extended.

The respiratory muscles also undergo spasm and respiration ceases. This may result in cyanosis which passes off as the spasm ceases. This phase lasts for a few seconds, seldom more than half a minute, and is followed by the clonic phase.

The *clonic phase* (alternate contraction and relaxation) is characterized by sharp, intermittent jerking movements of the voluntary muscles. These are powerful movements and may result in injuries such as dislocation of the shoulder or vertebral fractures; the tongue may be bitten. These convulsive movements may produce foaming at the mouth, and urine may be expelled. Incontinence of faeces is less common.

While consciousness is lost the pupils are dilated and do not react to light. Corneal and tendon reflexes may be lost and the plantar reflexes may be extensor for a short time.

During the *post-ictal phase* the patient may remain unconscious for a few seconds, or up to half an hour, and after recovery may sleep for several hours.

STATUS EPILEPTICUS

This phrase is used to describe the situation where one seizure follows another without an intervening period of consciousness. Unless this continuous train of fits ceases it may progress to a point where coma develops, damage due to brain hypoxia (lack of oxygen) becomes irreversible and hypercapnoea (excess of carbon dioxide in the blood) and death ensues.

This condition is a medical emergency and must be treated immediately (see below).

Some patients show a particular tendency to develop status epilepticus and should be identified as such so that they are given special attention if they have a seizure and are given intravenous or intramuscular diazepam (Valium) if a second seizure seems imminent.

ABSENCES OR PETIT MAL

Sometimes these episodes are called 'blank spells'. The subject stares into space and the eyes may roll up. All activity ceases for one or two seconds, after which it continues as if nothing had happened. The attacks are not usually associated with falling although this may occur, especially when the attacks are very numerous. (This is sometimes called akinetic epilepsy.) The EEG shows a very characteristic bilaterally synchronous high-amplitude three-per-second spike and wave discharges.

The presence of petit mal does not exclude the possibility of coexisting grand mal or the possibility that it might develop later.

COMPLEX PARTIAL SEIZURES (TEMPORAL LOBE EPILEPSY)

The clinical picture depends upon whether the epileptic discharge remains localized to the temporal areas or spreads throughout the brain to produce a major fit.

The forms taken by temporal lobe epilepsy may be exceedingly complex and may involve the following:

1. impairment of consciousness;
2. cognitive symptoms: episodes of forgetfulness;
3. affective symptoms: fear, laughter, depression, paranoia;
4. psychosensory symptoms: hallucinations, distortion of size, feelings of unreality (*jamais vu*) feelings of familiarity (*deja vu*);
5. psychomotor symptoms (automatisms): walking, undressing, chewing movements, aggressive behaviour.

FOCAL FITS (JACKSONIAN EPILEPSY)

This type of fit usually begins with movements of the thumb and index finger, angle of the mouth or great toe. As the seizure becomes more severe the movement spreads centrally and may involve both sides of the body when consciousness is lost.

MYOCLONIC FITS

A myoclonic spasm is a brief shock-like muscular contraction which may be very slight or extremely violent. There are a large number of conditions associated with this type of seizure and although the prevalence of myoclonic epilepsy is low in the general population it is much higher in the mentally handicapped, since it is often associated with degenerative brain disorders.

INFANTILE SPASMS

These appear during the first few months of life and consist of a sudden flexion of arms, head, neck and trunk with drawing up of the knees ('salaam' attacks).

The EEG shows a more or less continuous slow spike and wave activity which has been called hypsarrhythmia. The underlying pathology usually consists of a condition which produces widespread cerebral damage such as hypoglycaemia, phenyl-ketonuria or tuberous sclerosis.

The only treatment which, if used early enough, may arrest the process is ACTH or steroids.

As can be seen from the classification there are other forms of epilepsy but the forms described above will account for the majority of types seen in the mentally handicapped.

ELECTROENCEPHALOGRAPHY

All patients who are suspected of having epilepsy should have electroencephalography performed since it may help to elucidate the diagnosis and reveal other, possibly causative, pathology. It is always necessary to employ provocative stimuli such as over-breathing and photic stimulation since abnormalities may only be revealed in this way.

If there is sufficient evidence to make temporal lobe epilepsy a likely diagnosis it may be necessary to use special sphenoidal leads; this procedure involves the use of an anaesthetic.

It is important to bear in mind the limitations of this investigation. Most forms of epilepsy do not produce a pattern which is absolutely diagnostic and, indeed, an EEG without epileptic features does not exclude this diagnosis. Even the highly characteristic pattern of three-per-second spike and wave patterns may be associated with types of epilepsy other than petit mal. Equally, in grand mal there is no single characteristic pattern – there may be paroxysmal (periodic) diffuse multiple spikes or isolated outbursts of spikes or sharp wave activity.

If the facilities are available it may be possible to correlate particular forms of behaviour with abnormal EEG patterns. If absences can be shown to coincide with three-per-second spike and wave activity this would confirm the diagnosis and if unusual, repetitive mannerisms and/or behaviour disturbances can be shown to coincide with paroxysmal EEG abnormalities this would be an indication to use anticonvulsants. This picture is not so-called 'subclinical' epilepsy but one of the many atypical forms of epilepsy. Stereotypes however, are not associated with abnormal EEG activity. Clearly an abnormal EEG can only be interpreted in relation to the clinical history.

Special preparations must be made for the EEG recording with mentally handicapped persons. Many are afraid of the strange surroundings, the darkened room and the flashing lights. It is important that they be accompanied by one or two people they know and trust, and in many cases sedation may be necessary. If the subject becomes agitated while the electrodes are being placed, 10 mg of diazepam administered intravenously, and repeated if necessary, may be the only way in which an acceptable record can be obtained. Droperidol, either orally or by intramuscular injection, is also used in some departments. Suitable syringes, medication and easily removable (Velcro type) tourniquets should be at hand with an attendant who is able to give intravenous injections quickly and efficiently.

DIFFERENTIAL DIAGNOSIS

There are many conditions which may be confused with epilepsy and each of them may have numerous causes.

The many causes of fits in the very young are normally dealt with by paediatricians.

Differential diagnosis may be more difficult in the mentally handicapped because many of these patients may not be able to give a useful history.

Some of the conditions which it is important to exclude are listed below.

1. Breath-Holding Attacks

These may begin as a temper tantrum and go on to a breath-holding attack which may terminate in cyanosis, rigidity and convulsive movements.

There is almost always a precipitating cause which is associated with frustration or the need to gain attention. They will cease if totally ignored.

2. Simulated Seizures

Fits may be simulated by any patient including the severely retarded where the subject has presumably been reinforced in this behaviour by the reactive behaviour of those responsible for his care. Such fits may be very convincing, and the presence of injury does not exclude this diagnosis, although they hardly ever happen without an audience.

The onset of the attack is usually gradual and the subject does not lose consciousness. There are frequently vocalizations which may resemble the cry of grand mal but are more likely to be words, laughing or crying. Associated movements tend to be voluntary in type rather than tonic and then clonic, but the fit may be indistinguishable from grand mal or petit mal.

The corneal reflex is retained and attempts to open the eyes are accompanied by contraction of the muscles of the eyelid.

Occasionally, especially in the mentally handicapped, a simulated fit may be aborted by exhorting the subject to stop and do something else.

The fact that fits may be simulated by no means excludes the possibility that epilepsy and simulated fits may co-exist – indeed the presence of epilepsy makes this more likely.

3. Syncope

Syncopal attacks, for which there are many causes, consist of a transient loss of consciousness produced by a sudden reduction of blood-flow to the brain. Pallor, perspiration, slow pulse and flaccidity are distinguishing features and if anoxia is severe, transient rigidity and even twitching may occur. There may be incontinence if the bladder is full.

The period of unconsciousness is short (provided the patient's head is not held up) and confusion, sleep and automatism do not occur.

If a reliable history is available the diagnosis is usually not difficult.

4. Anxiety Attacks

In anxiety attacks consciousness is not lost and there is associated giddiness, palpitations and sweating at the onset. However, if the attack is accompanied by *hyperventilation*, this may be followed by syncope.

5. Nightmares

These may be presented as fits. Some parents may need to present

105

their children as physically ill, and it may be difficult to get them to accept that their child does not have epilepsy – even if the diagnosis of epilepsy is excluded by a period of inpatient observation.

6. Fits Associated with Drugs

In addition to provoking seizures phenothiazines may produce tardive dyskinesia (inability to move parts of the body) which may resemble focal epilepsy.

Consideration must also be given to the possibility that anticonvulsant drugs may have been withdrawn inadvertently or deliberately with resulting *withdrawal fits*.

8. Previous Misdiagnosis

Patients may have been on anticonvulsant drugs for many years without the diagnosis having been correctly made. Drug withdrawal must be gradual to avoid withdrawal fits and thus perpetuate the misdiagnosis.

9. Photosensitive Epilepsy

Photosensitive epilepsy, or television epilepsy, is always associated with a flickering light source. If the EEG is abnormal only during photic stimulation the only treatment that may be necessary is to ensure that the subject is more than 6 feet away from the television set.

10. Narcoleptic Attacks

These have all the features of natural sleep. There are no motor features and the patient is easily aroused.

11. Cataleptic Attacks

In contrast, during a cataleptic attack voluntary power is lost while consciousness is retained.

The tonic and clonic motor features of a grand mal attack together with the loss of consciousness, rapid pulse and anoxia will usually allow the diagnosis to be made with assurance.

AFTER THE DIAGNOSIS IS MADE

Once the diagnosis of epilepsy is confirmed it is necessary to discuss the management of the patient with parents, care staff and the patient. In practice it may be found necessary to repeat the explanations given several times, since most parents need confirmation of what is, for them, a new and shocking experience. They must be told that epilepsy *per se* is not likely to be the cause of the mental handicap, that epilepsy can be associated with intellectual levels from severe mental handicap to superior levels of intellect, and that both the epilepsy and the mental handicap are likely to be due to the same underlying brain damage.

It must be pointed out that it may be necessary to accept a certain number of fits and that it is important that the patient be lively and able to learn rather than over-sedated. If you outline the treatment programme, explain the difference between mental handicap, mental illness and epilepsy, show your own determination to improve matters, this is likely to improve family morale considerably.

It will be necessary to point out that while the treatment of epilepsy is the removal of the cause, this is very rarely possible.

Associated problems such as fear, shame and community acceptance should be brought up, if the family does not raise this issue. These factors do not necessarily feature in every family but if they do, it is important that they be discussed. (See Living with Epilepsy, P. 119.)

Parents should be advised that the patient should be allowed to lead as full a life as possible and should be encouraged to engage in physical activities as much as possible. Obviously pursuits such as climbing dangerous heights and cycling in traffic must be prohibited; but swimming is allowed if the patient is constantly accompanied by a skilled lifesaver.

The avoidance of such activities will not only impoverish the subject's life but is unlikely to alter the frequency of injuries since these may be equally severe in a domestic environment. In fact there is some evidence that the more general activity that is undertaken, and the more epileptics engage in tasks requiring concentration, the less likely they are to have fits.

Factors which may predispose to fits should be discussed with the family and efforts should be made to avoid or treat these as soon as they become apparent. The factors usually involved are infections, constipation, alterations in salt and water balance (fever, renal disorders, vomiting), and the effects of television or flashing lights of any kind.

The presence of epilepsy in a family member may precipitate a number of psychological phenomena which are basically similar to those seen when any shocking event occurs in a family, e.g. birth of severely mentally handicapped child.

Parents are often concerned that epilepsy may be genetically determined. They may usually be reassured that epilepsy in the mentally handicapped is mostly caused by cerebral lesions and that the epilepsy itself is unlikely to be hereditary in nature.

It is both impossible and unnecessary to guard against every risk, and where there is obvious overprotection this raises the same questions that overprotection involves in any family.

It is of the utmost importance that RECORDS of the fits be kept, since it is control of the severity and frequency of seizures that is the main object of management. Charts must not be made too complicated since they are less likely to be used and records which are not reliably kept will be misleading. The basic minimum of information required is the date and number of fits that have occurred and it may be necessary to be satisfied with this amount of information. It is, however, highly desirable to have a description of the fits as well. If informants are able and willing to perform this task, the difference between a description of the fit that was observed (e.g. unconsciousness, jerking movements, bitten tongue) and a diagnosis (e.g. grand mal) must be made. This distinction is important since different informants may offer different diagnoses while their observations are more likely to be consistent. Rarer or mixed types of epilepsy are more likely to be diagnosed in this way.

The chart is much more likely to be used reliably if it is hung on a board in a central position than if it is kept in notes or in a drawer.

MANAGEMENT

The treatment of epilepsy is concerned with the prevention of fits and no attempt should be made to abort or modify the isolated fit.

Prevention

This consists of correct medication, encouraging as normal a life as possible; treating febrile illnesses promptly and, if necessary, temporarily increasing drug dosages; avoiding hunger, thirst and constipation; and avoiding regular flashing lights, such as television sets and fluorescent tubes.

Management of the Fit

The management of the individual attack consists only of preventing the patient from injuring himself and ensuring a clear airway if this is obstructed. When a patient has a fit he should be:

1. Laid face down upon the ground with the head, which should not be raised, at right angles to the neck facing to one side to provide the best airway and allow saliva and vomit to escape and to prevent the tongue from falling back into the throat.
2. Removed from danger such as sharp objects, water, hot stoves or electrical appliances.
3. No attempt should be made to give anything by mouth. Usually there is not the time, nor is it desirable, to put a gag between the teeth. This manoeuvre may injure the teeth and great skill is needed in using it correctly.
4. If the patient is sleepy and/or confused after the fit no attempt should be made to arouse him but he should be allowed to rest quietly until fully conscious.

USE OF DRUGS

The aim of drug therapy is to reduce the frequency and severity of attacks while avoiding the undesirable effects of medication as much as possible.

With intractable forms of epilepsy the situation may be reached where the price for good control may be oversedation, and it may be wiser to accept more attacks and allow the patient to be more lively and in touch with his environment.

There are wide individual variations in responsiveness to anti-epileptic drugs and it is worth experimenting with different drugs if the response to a particular drug, given in dosages which ensure an adequate serum level, is unsatisfactory.

It must be explained to all concerned that once drug treatment has started it must be continued for 3 years after the attacks cease before consideration can be given to slowly withdrawing the drug. This is much less likely to happen in the mentally handicapped than in other epilepsies, and many mentally handicapped patients must be kept on anticonvulsants indefinitely, often with rather unsatisfactory control.

In patients with behaviour difficulties it may be useful to use a liquid preparation rather than tablets, to ensure that the medication is actually swallowed.

All the drugs used in the treatment of epilepsy have toxic effects and an awareness of these is particularly important in the handicapped, since many of them are unable to properly describe any unwanted side-effects which may occur.

For the same reason careful observation and follow-up is necessary. With all the drugs used particular care must be taken with the use of sedatives since their action will be potentiated by anticonvulsants. This effect is, of course, found with alcohol as well.

It seems that antidepressant drugs, as well as the major tranquilizers (particulary phenothiazines), lower the seizure threshold and may thus increase the number of fits. The co-existence of epilepsy and mental illness is not uncommon and it may, therefore, be necessary to reduce the dosage of antidepressant drugs and/or increase the dose of anticonvulsants.

Although particular drugs tend to have specific indications for use these are by no means rigid, and it may be necessary to experiment with several drugs until the most suitable is found.

Those responsible for administering anti-epileptic drugs must be warned not to change the dose without consultation and, in particular, not to stop the treatment because the fits have improved, since this may precipitate status epilepticus.

Table 7.1 Drug dosage and indications for use

Drug	Dosage	Recommended Use
Phenytoin (Epanutin)	*Adults and children:* start with 2–400 mg/day, up to 600 mg/day.	Grand mal; focal epilepsy
Sodium valproate (Epilim)	Start with 600 mg/day in divided doses and slowly build up to optimal dose. Maximum is 2600 mg/day. *Children:* 20–30 mg/kg $^{-1}$/day $^{-1}$.	Petit mal; focal epilepsy; grand mal
Carbamazepine (Tegretol)	*Adults:* start 1–200 mg twice daily, increasing slowly to best response; 1200 mg may be needed. *Children:* 2 to 5 X 200 mg/day.	Focal epilepsy; grand mal
Clonazepam (Rivotrol)	Start *Adults:* 1 mg/day *Children:* 0.5 mg/day Slowly increased to optimal control.	Myoclonic epilepsy; grand mal; focal epilepsy; petit mal
Ethosuximide (Zerontin) (Emeside)	Start with 2 X 250 mg/day. Slow increments until control obtained; up to 2 g/day.	Petit mal
Phenobarbitone• (Luminal phenobarbitone spansules)	30–300 mg/day in divided doses.	See note below

•Phenobarbitone (Luminal): at one time this was the drug of first choice in the treatment of all forms of epilepsy but in view of its serious drawbacks and the advantages of newer drugs it has virtually no place in the current treatment of epilepsy.

It very frequently causes drowsiness when used in effective doses and often produces restlessness, overactivity and disturbed behaviour, especially in children. Other side-effects are vertigo, headaches, nausea, ataxia and delirium. It may also be habit-forming.

It affects the metabolism of other drugs, particularly anticonvulsants and steroids including the contraceptive pill. This may result in these compounds being reduced to ineffective concentrations in the serum.

ANTICONVULSANT SERUM LEVELS

Now that the routine estimation of the level of anticonvulsant drugs in the blood can be done it has become possible to establish the upper levels at which they are likely to produce toxic effects, and the lower levels at which the amount of drug available is unlikely to be sufficient to suppress fits. Where this service is available close monitoring of serum levels has allowed a more rational approach to drug usage with consequent improved control of fits. Serum level estimations have shown that most anticonvulsant drugs remain in the serum for sufficiently long periods of time to allow administration no more frequently than twice a day. This is a great convenience since it avoids the difficulties associated with the midday dose.

Control of dosage with the help of serum level estimations has become the preferred method of management because the relationship between the oral dose of drug – even when calculated according to body weight – and the serum level is rather poor. The great individual variation between patients and, indeed, in the same patient from time to time, is due to many factors including differences in absorption, binding to serum proteins, and increased rates of destruction which may be due to drugs such as barbiturates and phenytoin; these of course, are themselves used in the treatment of epilepsy.

Nevertheless, serum levels should only be used as a guide since it is the frequency and severity of fits that should be the main determinant of the manner of drug administration.

Table 7.1 summarizes the dosage and indications for use of some of the most commonly used drugs in the treatment of epilepsy. It is important to emphasize that the range of dosage is very wide and those given are only a rough guide: the optimal dose should be determined by estimation of blood levels, the degree of seizure control and the presence of toxic effects.

DRUGS USED IN THE TREATMENT OF EPILEPSY

Phenytoin (Epanutin)

The early side-effects of phenytoin include nausea, nervousness, weight loss and unsteadiness. These early effects usually subside with continued use.

With prolonged usage other toxic effects may appear such as blood disorders, hypertrophy of the gums, excessive hair growth on the face and body, coarsening of features, excessive motor activity and various types of mental disturbance.

The first signs of *overdosage* are ataxia, dysarthria and nystagmus.

Phenytoin levels may be elevated by other drugs, such as antituberculous agents, disulfiram, dicoumarol anticoagulants, sulthiam and pheneturide.

Phenytoin is a drug which exhibits the saturation phenomenon, i.e. at lower serum concentrations there is a more or less linear relationship between dosage and serum level, but as the serum level increases there is a very sudden increase in the serum concentration which may then reach toxic levels very quickly. For example an incremental dose of only 50 mg may be enough to increase the serum level from $10 \mu g/ml$ to toxic levels.

Consequently incremental doses of this drug should become progressively smaller as the serum concentration increases. The 25 mg capsule is useful under these circumstances.

When the liquid form of phenytoin is used it is essential that the bottle be thoroughly shaken whenever it is administered, since the active drug tends to settle. If this is not done the first samples will have low concentrations of the drug and the later ones will have excessive amounts.

Carbamezepine (Tegretol)

This is the drug of first choice in focal epilepsies. The commonest side-effects are generalized rashes which may be light-sensitive. There are other more serious side-effects but they are rare.

Sodium Valproate (Epilim)

This drug potentiates the action of monoamine oxidase inhibitors and other antidepressants. It is eliminated partly as ketones in the urine and may thus produce false-positive results in diabetics.

Among the side-effects of valproate are transient hair loss, tremor and thrombocytopenia.

Clonazepam (Rivotril)

This drug often reduces the incidence of myoclonic attacks where other drugs have failed. Like Valium and Mogadon it is a benzodiazepine derivative and can be used intravenously in the treatment of status epilepticus. In this case the 1 mg ampoule must be diluted with an equal amount of water immediately before use and given by slow intravenous injection. If used in a drip 3 mg may be diluted in 250 ml of normal saline, dextrose or dextrose/saline.

After prolonged usage fits may recur while the patient is still on the drug and the dose may have to be increased or another drug substituted.

It must be administered in three or four doses during 24 hours since it has a relatively short serum half-life.

When used with other drugs such as phenytoin or phenobarbitone it may produce toxic effects at a relatively lower dosage.

The side-effects include drowsiness, weakness and disturbances of co-ordination. These occur early in treatment and tend to disappear in time. In infants and children clonazepam may give rise to the troublesome side-effects of salivary or bronchial hypersecretion.

Ethosuximide (Zarontin)

This drug is only used in the treatment of petit mal, and may be used in combination with other drugs in intractable cases.

Side-effects include drowsiness, depression, ataxia, anorexia, nausea and vomiting.

CONTROL OF MEDICATION

The current approach to drug therapy is to choose a single drug and adjust the dose to maintain the optimal blood-level. If, after several months, it is felt that the control of fits could be improved upon, the addition of a second drug might be considered. If satisfactory control is obtained then the patient is followed up in the usual way.

If it is decided to withdraw the first drug because of unacceptable side-effects this should be done gradually over several weeks.

Similar caution should be exercised when it has been decided to embark upon a trial of complete drug withdrawal. This is normally considered if there have been no fits for 3 years.

Clearly, if fits start again when the dose is reduced it will be necessary to return to the previous dosage schedule and maintain this for a further period of 3 years. The reason for this cautious approach is that the sudden withdrawal of medication may lead to status epilepticus.

Treatment of Overdose of Anticonvulsant Drugs

Where the side-effects of these drugs become unacceptable, merely reducing the dose or stopping the drug temporarily and then starting again at a lower dose will usually suffice. If, however, there has been a large overdose and coma threatens or the patient is actually unconscious, the following regime is indicated:

1. Aspiration of the gastric contents.
2. Maintenance of the airway – either with a simple airway or with an endotracheal tube if the gag reflex is absent.
3. Routine temperature, pulse, respiration and blood pressure readings (at 15 min intervals).
4. Administration of oxygen, either with a standard plastic mask or via an endotracheal tube by an anaesthetist or other suitably trained person.
5. If convulsions occur a muscle relaxant should be used and artificial ventilation should be instituted.
6. Haemodialysis, exchange transfusion or alkaline diuresis have been successfully used.

The Ketogenic Diet

In epilepsy which is unresponsive to other measures, the use of a ketogenic diet may be useful. This diet contains a very high proportion of fats and oils. It is expensive, difficult to manage and somewhat unpalatable, at least in the early stages of its use. It is less effective in pure petit mal or temporal lobe seizures, its principal indication being in myoclonic epilepsy.

The most practical approach in the use of this diet is to introduce it gradually and give the parents and/or patient several written copies of the diet sheet. The hospital dietitian should be part of the management team when this treatment is used.

Management of Status Epilepticus

Status epilepticus is the condition where one seizure follows another without an intervening period of full consciousness. This is a dangerous, even life-threatening situation and unless this succession of fits is stopped the patient may suffer brain damage from anoxia, develop high temperatures and may die from cardio-respiratory failure.

Some patients, particularly among the severely subnormal, have a particular tendency to develop status epilepticus.

If a second fit starts without an intervening period of consciousness:

Diazepam (Valium) 10 mg as a suppository per rectum should be given. (This is the simplest form of treatment and is very effective.)

Alternatively diazepam (Valium) may be given intravenously 5–15 mg by slow infusion, judging the dose against the clinical response.

The intravenous injection must be given slowly over 2–3 min to avoid respiratory depression. If the patient does not respond rapidly it may become necessary to use an intravenous drip of diazepam in normal saline or glucose running at the rate of 10 mg/15 min (maximum dose: 3 mg/kg body-weight over 24 h).

This mixture must be prepared freshly for each occasion and no other drugs must be added to the infusion.

In intractable cases the insertion of a cuffed endotracheal tube and the use of additional oxygen is necessary to protect against inhaling saliva or vomit and to prevent oxygen deprivation. The disadvantage of using paraldehyde is that it may cause abscesses when given intramuscularly and phlebitis when given intravenously.

If an intravenous drip is necessary the patient should be cared for in an intensive care unit since the risk of respiratory depression may necessitate the use of artificial ventilation.

There is evidence which suggests that there is an increase in benzodiazepine receptors after seizures; the resulting increase in sensitivity to this anticonvulsant may explain its effectiveness in status epilepticus.

Petit mal status may be treated by ethosuccimide 250 mg/kg or, preferably, sodium valproate (Epilim) 200 mg/kg, since petit mal status is not dangerous and sodium valproate is rapidly absorbed from the stomach. It is available in liquid form.

Drug Non-Compliance

That patients will receive their medication as instructed cannot always be taken for granted, since the presence of an epileptic child in a family may be associated with a wide spectrum of family psychopathology.

At one extreme are parents who, consciously or unconsciously, wish to have their child institutionalized and, therefore, make the illness worse by giving anticonvulsants in an erratic fashion or not at all. There are others, staff and parents, who have an antipathy to any form of medication and feel they should stop it as soon as possible. On the other hand there are the parents who have an over-investment in their child and cannot bear the thought of it growing up to independence. This form of interaction is one facet of the larger problem of infantilization, i.e. the creation of a state of perpetual dependence upon the parent. The presence of epilepsy in a member of the family may signify him in the role of scape-goat or he may be the object of various forms of family manipulation.

These problems are notoriously difficult to deal with and admission is often advisable as a preliminary to a change in the family dynamics.

If admission is seen to be necessary this should be insisted upon in a firm manner, since many families may be reluctant to part with their children because of the feelings of guilt involved. Under these circumstances it is the duty of the professional worker involved to take the 'blame' of admission upon himself and thereby remove some of it from the family. If they complain that admission was insisted upon more or less against their wishes the professional worker will have to carry this blame with as good a grace as possible, bearing in mind that if the family did not really want to part with their child they would not have done so; in any case they can insist on having him home at any time.

PROGNOSIS

The likelihood that fits will be completely suppressed is small, particularly in the more severely handicapped, since they are more likely to have more of the adverse prognostic factors listed below.

Duration of Epilepsy

The longer a patient has been having seizures, in spite of adequate treatment, the less likely is he to respond well in the long term. Various workers have produced evidence which suggests that vigorous anticonvulsant treatment at the onset of the condition can reduce later seizure frequency.

Type of Seizure and Presence of more than One Seizure Type

Pure petit mal in non-brain-damaged individuals tends to improve with age, but if it is combined with other types of seizures the prognosis is much poorer. Mixed fits of any kind are generallly more difficult to control both in the short and longer term.

Seizure Frequency and Severity

The more frequent and severe the fits, in spite of adequate medication, the poorer the prognosis. In particular, if fits occur in *clusters*, with relatively fit-free periods in between (the so-called 'long-range rhythm') and especially if the clusters have episodes of status epilepticus, the less likely is it that good control can be achieved.

Associated Neurological Features

Patients with brain damage do not respond to treatment as well as those in whom there is no evidence of coarse brain disease. Structural damage associated with epilepsy is found in many conditions seen in the severely mentally handicapped.

Electroencephalographic Patterns

If the EEG is grossly abnormal, with widespread high-voltage sharp-wave activity the likelihood of fits continuing is greater.

Where mental handicap is associated with epilepsy both states are likely to be due to the same underlying pathology. However, anticonvulsant drugs have also been incriminated as a factor in poor cognitive functioning, the percentage varying from 15% (when bromides and phenobarbitone were commonly used) to 5% (more recently). It has been shown that phenobarbitone, diphenylhydantoin and ethosuccimides are all capable of causing mental slowing, impaired concentration, psychiatric disorders and speech disturbance. Nevertheless the correct use of drugs may result in a *net* improvement of learning if fits are better controlled.

LIVING WITH EPILEPSY

Since epilepsy is a chronic condition which may change in its manifestations it is essential that the management of the patient is an ongoing process with regular visits by the family. On these occasions the following factors must be considered:

1. The frequency and severity of the fits. The parents should be asked to keep a simple diary as a record. This record should be examined in detail.
2. Possible precipitating and alleviating factors.
3. The manner in which the family is adjusting to the problem.
4. The manner in which the patient is coping with work or school, leisure and his social activities.
5. Changes in temperament – particularly with respect to irritability and behaviour disturbances.
6. The patient should be examined for changes in the gums, skin and mental state.
7. Periodic estimations of drug levels, serum calcium and serum folate should be done.

All of the advice and explanation given to the family will have to be repeated several times, because it is unfamiliar and associated with a disorder with unpleasant emotional connotations and, as with most forms of reassurance, this must also be reinforced at regular intervals. The family need to be told that the child will not die because of a fit, that he does not need 24-hour surveillance and that he should not be spoiled because he has epilepsy.

The parents should be encouraged to join a voluntary organisation where many of their emotional and practical problems may be alleviated by their involvement with other families having similar experiences.

References

Eyman, R. K., Capes, L., Moore, B. C. and Zacholfsky, T. Retardates with seizures. *Am. J. Ment. Defic.*, **74**, 651

Corbett, J. A. and Harris, R. (1964). *Epilepsy in Children with Severe Mental Handicap*. Symposium no. 16. (London: Institute for Research into Mental and Multiple Handicap)

8

SENSORY HANDICAPS

G. B. Simon

In this chapter the terms blind, deaf and deaf/blind are used repeatedly but it must not be assumed that the subjects are necessarily totally blind, deaf or deaf/blind. In a review of deaf/blind units in several parts of the world, Myers (1976), reported that less than 10% in these units were totally blind and deaf. The majority are, therefore, likely to have some remnant of either or of both senses, and one of the purposes of this chapter is to alert everyone involved with such individuals to the importance of discovering this, so that the patients may be trained to use their residual senses. If the subject is also mentally handicapped, this is even more important, as it is more than likely that without the appropriate stimulation and training these sensory remnants will never be used.

INCIDENCE

The results of a survey in Wessex mentioned in *Better Services for the Mentally Handicapped* (1971), indicated that among severely mentally handicapped children in hospital, 1 in 5 had defects of vision or hearing and 1 in 20 was blind; amongst the adults 1 in 5 had defects of vision or hearing. The most recent report of the Development Team for the Mentally Handicapped (1979) states that based on the reports received from staff, 1 in 5 of the children, and 1 in 10 of adults in hospital suffer from defects of vision and hearing. The total number in hospitals is in the region of 50 000. Tempowski *et al.* (1974) reported that among 1049 referrals to an assessment clinic for the mentally handicapped 145 (34 adults and 111 children), or over 13%, were diagnosed as deaf with losses over 30 dB. Balkany *et al.* (1978) found a binaural hearing loss over 15 dB in 64% of adults suffering from Down's syndrome.

Despite some variations in the findings of these studies, possibly due to varying criteria and method, all report a significant number of mentally handicapped with disabilities of hearing and vision.

ASSESSMENT OF HEARING AND VISION

The presence of sensory handicaps will influence any developmental training programme and, therefore, steps to detect them must be an essential part of early assessment so that they can be alleviated if possible. It is also necessary that everyone associated with training should be aware of the extent of any disability, and take it into account in training programmes.

Knowledge and experience of the detection and management of these handicaps in children and adults of average intelligence is now considerable, but where the severely mentally handicapped are concerned it remains very limited. As a result of this a significant number of mentally handicapped adults and children with additional sensory handicaps are frequently regarded as far more retarded than they really are.

It is also fairly common to find that, through a lack of appropriate early treatment and management, under-functioning, both mentally and physically, can occur. In addition there may be behaviour problems, psychotic features and other psychiatric disturbances; these can make detection of the disability, and management, even more difficult.

It is therefore all the more important for every assessment procedure to include an investigation of hearing and vision.

SIMPLE TESTS OF VISION AND HEARING

Sections of a simple method for assessment of the senses are reproduced below. These are taken from *The Next Step on the Ladder*, by permission of the British Institute of Mental Handicap.

Sight

The following simple tests are designed to find out how the individual reacts visually to near objects and activities. Test objects should be held at 6 ft (2 m) initially and the distance reduced until a response is obtained, or it is clear that none is likely. Although a light is usually easier to see, for a visually handicapped individual, than is some other object, some children will find the latter more interesting. The first four stages listed below will indicate whether the person focuses on an object and is able to follow its movement. The next two stages assess the ability to discriminate objects.

1. Turns head and eyes towards light.
2. Follows light moved slowly in front of face.
3. Watches object moved in line of vision.
4. Follows object moved in front of face.
5. Searches for a 10 mm (or ⅜ in.) diameter sweet, or similar-sized object, held in palm of tester's hand.
6. Locates the object from amongst others of similar size and shape; for example, cube, round object, or small coin.

Hearing

In all the tests that follow, start at a distance of 6 ft (2 m) and gradually bring the sound closer until a reaction is obtained; if none occurs at 1 ft (30 cm) from the ear, it must be assumed, for all practical purposes, that there is no response.

1. Shows awareness, through a movement, twitch or other reaction, to a drum beat at 6 ft (2 m) or less.
2. Stills at familiar sound, e.g. voice, music, toy rattle.
3. Turns in direction of sound.
4. Shows appreciation of tone of voice, e.g. anger or praise.

5. Understands simple spoken instructions, e.g. 'sit down'.
6. Understands more complex instructions, e.g. 'put the spoon in the cup'.

PROGRAMMES: ENCOURAGE LOOKING AND LISTENING

If some sight or hearing is evident then it will be necessary to encourage the use of it, as many mentally handicapped individuals have never been taught to use their residual senses. This is also advisable where no responses have been obtained, as this may be due to previous habitual lack of usage.

Looking can be encouraged during any activity by holding objects in front of the individual, and as close as necessary, in various positions, so that the subject must reach out to hold it, rather than having it placed in his hand. As progress is made, the individual can be asked questions appropriate to his general level of function, such as where objects are, what they are, what colour they are, what they look like, and so on.

Listening should be encouraged during all activity; for example, by making a noise with an object such as tapping it on the table, or by tapping a spoon in a cup to direct the person's attention to it; by talking and describing what is going to happen; by asking simple questions which only require a 'Yes' or 'No' or an appropriate sign in reply, such as 'Do you want this cup of tea now?' rather than simply placing a cup of tea in front of him or feeding it to him. *Note*: Should an individual be suspected of suffering from a deficit of sight or hearing as a result of these tests and stimulation, he or she should be referred for further advice from a specialist consultant so that any possible remedial measures may be taken.

Training

Programmes to increase communication, increase self-help and change behaviour referred to elsewhere in this book are equally applicable to those with sensory handicaps but may need adaptation to overcome any sensory defects. It is suggested that *The Next Step on the Ladder* is among the most useful, as each step in this assessment is accompanied by a simple programme to help parents and staff, who may have had little or no experience of these problems, to carry them out. There are forms of developmental assessment which provide a 'social quotient' standardized for blind children in existence; among these one of the most widely used is the *Social Maturity Scale for Blind Pre-School Children* by Maxfield and Bucholz (1957).

EARLY ADVICE AND GUIDANCE TO PARENTS

Using Residual Senses

The needs for parents of handicapped children to be given support, advice and assistance in acceptance immediately after birth is no less urgent or imperative for children who suffer from a sensory handicap. In addition, however, because most human beings have such a highly developed sense of hearing and vision, both of which function at a distance, the parents are less aware of the needs of a child with deficiencies in these areas. The very close physical contact of the cat with its newborn kittens, or the dog with its puppies, does not typify human behaviour after the first few days or during breast-feeding. Babies with normal senses will themselves very soon learn to use these senses to establish contact with those around them, and will soon begin to anticipate pleasurable activities such as the approach of mother, by the sound of her footsteps and voice, and will very quickly recognize her from across the room. Emotions and moods can be conveyed by sounds and looks which the young normal child soon learns to appreciate.

All these natural occurrences assist in development; the child enjoys what he sees and hears; he raises his head, sits up, stands and ultimately tries to walk in order to increase experience and pleasure. The stimulus for much of the child's behaviour and development is the result of what he sees and hears. If, however, the world of the child without normal vision and/or hearing can be imagined, it should not be difficult to appreciate its difficulties. An hypothesis of how compensation occurs in humans (Mykelbust, 1966) provides a useful guide to parents and other. It is as follows:

Handicap	Order in which other senses compensate
Deaf	Sight – Touch – Smell – Taste
Hard of hearing	Sight – Residual hearing – Touch – Smell – Taste
Deaf/blind	Touch – Smell – Taste
Partially sighted	Hearing – Residual vision – Touch – Smell – Taste
Blind	Hearing – Touch – Smell – Taste

Thus mother must get close to her baby, encourage it to touch the face it cannot see, feel the movements of lips in speaking, and the vibrations of the voice it does not hear. Brothers, sisters and other children are frequently the best aids to development, once they are told of the child's problems, as they are less inhibited about closeness and behaviour which may be unconventional in a sighted, hearing world. A simple handbook for parents, *Some Facts and Hints on Management* . . . is available from the British Institute of Mental Handicap. Freeman (1975) also wrote a very useful account of her own experiences and difficulties, together with advice on overcoming them.

Gestures to Indicate Needs

Children should be encouraged to use simple natural gestures to indicate their needs: food, drink, toilet, etc. A simple set of some 15 to 20 gestures is provided in diagrammatic form in the handbook mentioned above. All gestures should be accompanied by the equivalent spoken word in a loud, clear voice.

PROVISIONS FOR EDUCATION AND TRAINING

Children

Schools for children who have defects of vision and hearing and are of average or near-average intelligence, now exist in most parts of the world. However, most such services are still scarce while those for the combined deaf/blind disability are rarities and will probably continue to be so for some time. Similar facilities for those who are also mentally handicapped are almost non-existent.

For many of these children when placements are available they are frequently away from home in residential special schools or hospital units. Consequently, when they reach school-leaving age and must be placed locally, no suitable facility is available. They are, therefore, more often than not, left at home all day or placed in the nearest hospital for the mentally handicapped. Both these placements must be regarded as a retrograde step after 5 or more years at a school.

There are several internationally known voluntary organizations for the blind and deaf/blind which are increasingly becoming involved in education and training. A list of these is provided at the end of this chapter, and readers seeking more information should write to the appropriate address.

Adults

As indicated above, adult mentally handicapped people suffering from severe degrees of sensory handicap are generally even more deprived of facilities than children.

In the United Kingdom, with this deficiency in mind, the Department of Health and Social Security has sponsored a research project, through the British Institute of Mental Handicap, to look into the needs of the adolescent and adult visually handicapped. It is hoped this will produce a detailed form of developmental assessment and programmes associated with each step in this scale, thus enabling parents and relatively inexperienced staff to approach training in a constructive manner.

HOSTEL AND OTHER PROVISIONS

Most of the hostels and group homes for the blind and/or deaf in the United Kingdom are at present provided through voluntary associations for the blind or deaf. These are very limited, especially for adults, and where placements are likely to be needed, early enquiry should be made to the appropriate agency so that help is available when it is required.

Because of the scarcity of such provisions and of trained staff in the community, it is virtually impossible for hospitals to discharge many mentally handicapped patients who suffer from deafness or blindness, in spite of the fact that they may have improved through specialized training and teaching. It is now generally accepted that

127

many can reach a level of competence through the use of special aids and manual methods of communication, thus making hospital placement, or being left at home all day, quite inappropriate.

THE NEEDS OF FAMILIES

Parents will frequently wish to continue caring for their deaf/blind son or daughter, and to enable them to do this they must be provided with some basic instruction so that they can communicate with the child and continue the programmes followed during the day at a school or other centre.

Families will also require regular relief from the heavy burden of care which this places on them, and the short-term care, advocated elsewhere in this book, for the mentally handicapped should also be available to them. Unfortunately, the fact that a child or adult is blind, deaf, or both, makes the staff of ordinary hostels reluctant to accept them.

TRAINING FOR STAFF

The reluctance to accept people with such sensory and mental handicaps in existing centres and hostels can be overcome by providing some of the staff of these establishments with training and experience, through visits to the specialized schools and units which accommodate them, and by enabling staff to attend courses which will provide them with enough basic knowledge of management to enable them to cope.

In addition to the suggested staff visits to schools and units already working with the blind and deaf, and to residential workshops, there is now also the possibility of utilizing the travelling workshops organized by the British Institute of Mental Handicap.

Apart from the need for care-staff in hospitals for the mentally handicapped and elsewhere to become experienced in day-to-day management, there is also a need for more social workers to acquire experience and training in communication with patients through the use of hand signs.

References

Balkany, T. J. *et al.* (1979). Hearing loss in Down's syndrome. *Clinical Paediatrics*, **18**, 2 Feb.

Better Services for the Mentally Handicapped (1971). Command Paper 4683. (London: HMSO.)

Development Assessment and Programming for Blind and Blind/Deaf Adolescents and Adults. (British Institute of Mental Handicap; In press)

Development Team for the Mentally Handicapped (1979). *Second Report, 1978-1979.* (London: HMSO)

Freeman, P. (1975). *Understanding the Deaf/Blind Child.* (London: William Heinemann Ltd.)

Maxfield, K. E. and Bucholz, S. (1975). *Social Maturity Scale for Blind Pre-School Children.* (New York: American Foundation for the Blind,, Inc., 15 West 16th Street)

Myers, S. O. (1976). *Services for the Deaf/Blind.* (6th International Seminar of the Deaf/Blind, Sydney, Australia.)

Myklebust, H. R. (1966). *The Psychology of Deafness.* (Grune & Stratton)

The Next Step on the Ladder, rev. edn. (1980) (Kidderminster: British Institute of Mental Handicap)

Robbins, N. and Stenquist, G. (1967). *The Deaf-Blind Rubella Child.* (Watertown, Massachusetts, USA.) (Perkins School for the Blind)

Some Facts and Hints on Management to Parents of Young Children Suffering from Handicaps of Vision and/or Hearing. (Kidderminster: British Institute of Mental Handicap)

Tempowski, I., Felstead, F. and Simon, G. B. (1974). Deafness and the mentally retarded. *Apex*, vol. 2, no. 2

Further information is available from the following

The National Association for Deaf/Blind and Rubella Handicapped.
164 Cromwell Lane, Coventry, CV4 8AP.
> Publications on Deaf/Blind services, information to parents and others on management (formerly known as the Rubella Parents' Association).

The National Deaf Children's Society.
31 Gloucester Place, London W1.
> Publications dealing with problems of deafness for parents and others.

The Royal National Institute for the Blind.
224-6-8 Great Portland Street, London W1.
> Publications on the care, training, management and needs of the blind, designed to assist parents and staff.

The Royal National Institute for the Deaf.
105 Gower Street, London WC1.
> Publications covering every aspect of deafness and information.

9

MOTOR HANDICAP

D. M. Ricks

Anyone faced with the task of helping a profoundly physically handicapped retarded child is usually so impressed with the magnitude of the child's disabilities that he does not know where to start. Later he may be so disheartened by the child's slow response that he sees no point in persevering. It is to such a task that this chapter is addressed: to sketch out programmes the aims of which are to improve as much as possible postural control, hand-use and mobility, respecting the child's need to develop these by putting each skill to use in his own way. The objective is a more contented and exploratory child as well as a more efficiently functioning one.

TWO FORMS OF MOTOR HANDICAP: RETARDED AND CEREBRAL PALSIED CHILDREN

There are degrees of physical handicap in retarded children varying from the immobile child, unable to sit or even roll, who may neither look nor listen, to the active child with problems of gait and balance. The position of any given child on this spectrum will depend not only on the severity of his handicap but also on age and the level of care and stimulation enjoyed. The emphasis in this chapter will be on the younger, most severely handicapped child,

131

since these present the most daunting prospect (Cunningham and Sloper, 1978). It is helpful to distinguish two groups of such children: one with severe motor delay resulting from gross mental retardation (retarded group); the other with motor disorder due to brain damage involving the motor cortex, associated nuclei and pathways who will also function as retarded children (cerebral palsy group). The first impress one as being apathetic with poor social response; as having low/normal muscle tone. They often have poor head control, particularly when young, but if the head is moved, its position does not affect the tone of the limbs or the posture they adopted. These children often have little spontaneous movement, but when they choose are able to move symmetrically, i.e. both right and left limbs through the full range, often using both arms or legs together. They tend not to rotate their trunk, but turn, as it were, all in one piece; when held up or when attempting to sit or stand, they flex at hips and knees. The second group are a complete contrast. They are more alert and responsive, stiff rather than floppy, and are characterized by making strenuous efforts to move; these movements are usually asymmetrical and mis-directed or lead to spasm. This spasm is vulnerable to the position of the head: for instance if it is tilted back, shoulders retract and the trunk extends. Whatever his intention, the child's efforts may be distorted by reflex postures such as atonic neck reflexes which compel him, on turning his head, to extend the limb to which his face turns and flex the opposite limbs. These distorted movements result from the inability of the child's damaged cortex to inhibit or control reflex patterns. Similarly a lack of this inhibitory control prevents the child damping down his responses. These are therefore exaggerated with excitement or agitation, or even if the child tries hard when making a movement.

In general the motor handicap of the first group of children is a consequence of their general retardation so that they present basically a problem of learning. It is as if in their apathy they see no point in moving, and become stiffer, less mobile and more flexed so that more effort is needed to make any response. This in its turn promotes less stimulation from parents or staff around them. The fundamental principle of treatment for this group is to encourage motivation and movement experience. The second group of

Table 9.1 Distinctive responsiveness in the two forms of motor handicap

Features	Retarded group	Cerebral palsy group
History	May or may not have history of cerebral brain damage	History of cerebral (brain) damage
Appearance and response	Apathy: low motivation, slow eye movements, poor visual fixing. Little 'startle' reaction	Alert, excitable. Active eye movements. Interested visual following. 'Hair-trigger' reaction to 'startle'
Spontaneous movement	Little movement and little effort. Symmetrical limb use but total pattern	More movement and makes efforts. Asymmetrical limb-use e.g. arms more than legs; left more than right
Range of movement	Full range available, elicited by passive movement	Limited: often made more restricted by passive movement, e.g. in examination
Resting tone	Low/normal	Very low (ataxic). High (spastic)
Active tone	Sluggish, slow rise	Rapid rise, with tendency to spasm
Pattern of movement	'Primitive', e.g. both arms or legs moved together. Not affected by head position. Tendency to flex. Poor trunk rotation	Reflex pattern, greatly affected by position of head in space or on trunk. Frequent radiating associated movements with effort or excitement

children have difficulties in movement resulting from cerebral palsy. The implication is that their difficulties are the result of some insult or accident to what may have been a normal brain in presumably a normally motivated child. Treatment is aimed primarily at retaining the child's exploratory interest and enthusiasm to move, but to help bring it under his control to protect him from the frustration he must feel in his inability to direct and grade his motor efforts.

DISTINCTIVE RESPONSIVENESS IN THE TWO GROUPS

Distinguishing these groups of children is valuable because it directs attention to a fundamental contrast not only in the type of child and his disabilities but in the basic policy which governs his treatment programme. However in both cases we must always remember that we are dealing with the child as a person, so how to help him move more efficiently will depend not only on his disability and how we treat it, but also on his response to us and the world around him. There is some danger in regarding him as simply a motor problem, and even more to emphasize the need for him to move as normally as possible, when in fact how he sees himself, directs his attention and enjoys his world may be of much greater importance. Treatment should be aimed at equipping him to move as best he can in response to these interests.

An appreciation of the way such children are likely to react to parents or staff helping them is as important as an understanding of the basic aims of their therapy. The first group, the retarded children, need constant stimulation, and since they are so slow and unresponsive everyone helping them needs support to retain their enthusiasm (Scott, 1979). They need, too, to be helped to keep realistic perspectives, appreciating small gains however long in coming. The second group, the cerebral palsied children, are quite different since their responses are hair-trigger and the children may frequently be excitable or irritable. The problem for staff here is to help in a consistent and predictable way so that the child himself is able thereby to respond in a more calm, controlled manner, to keep his tone within limits and movements more graded.

RESULTING CONTRASTS IN GENERAL PRINCIPLES OF MANAGEMENT/TREATMENT

Thus the general treatment principles for each group have a different emphasis. The first group of retarded children need to be helped through a sequence of skills, each of which may be slow in appearing. Every effort must be made to be alert for any sign the child himself makes of initiating movement or taking visual interest in acquiring these skills, such as beginning to look or to roll or to reach. For these children it is vital that all staff are sensitive to, and capitalize on, the slightest change, respecting the child's own efforts and indeed his own tactics in reaching these aims, and

134

encouraging him in these efforts. This is not the type of child in whom one can insist on normal patterns of movement any more than one can successfully wait for the child to produce these skills spontaneously. The whole programme depends on finding means of motivating the child to raise his tone, to focus and sustain his interest, to improve his trunk rotation, and to respect his own ways of doing this, since the fundamental aim is to cultivate his spontaneity. With a cerebral palsy child such sustained pressure would be disastrous. For him, too, there are general principles of management, such as helping him stabilize his head by working bimanually in the mid-line, securing stable sitting and improved trunk control, and, as his motor skills develop, trying without too much confrontation to overcome or minimize bad habits of movement. All these should be pursued in a quiet, equable situation.

Table 9.2 Contrasts in general principles of management/treatment in two forms of motor handicap

N.B.   Each child is an individual: respect his interests and dislikes

Retarded group	*Cerebral palsy group*
1 Motivate, stimulate interest. Cultivate any spontaneity	Encourage and retain interest. Equip him to express spontaneity
2. Excite to raise tone	Teach? Coax? to grade tone
3. Encourage stimulation from the side and thereby trunk rotation	Concentrate on stimulation from front to keep head in mid-line and reduce asymmetrical reflex patterning
4. Needs lively motor experience: aim at exciting novel situation to initiate movement, however executed. Can improve and modify with practice	Aim at quite predictable situation with carefully graduated encouragement to reduce spasm and enable child to *control* own readily initiated movement
5. Uphold staff or parent morale to persevere. Difficult to keep going, with such slow return from child	Curb staff or parent impatience at variable response and achievement. Beware: 'He could do it if he tried harder' or 'if he feels like it'
6. Get him interested to make an effort	Keep him calm to keep trying

135

A TREATMENT PROGRAMME FOR THE RETARDED GROUP

Stages in the treatment of the retarded group of children would follow a particular sequence depending on the age and severity of the child's handicap. Assuming that he is an apathetic, totally unresponsive, helpless child, unable to sit or weight-bear, then priority must be given to establishing visual interest. It will be important to assess as carefully as possible whether the child's eyes and ears are functioning. This will mean obtaining pupil-responses, and necessitate an ophthalmological assessment, looking for lens opacities and retinal or fundal changes. It will need, too, a similar assessment of the child's ears, though here it may be necessary to resort to recording techniques to discover whether the child does hear. Nevertheless the child's ears should be recurrently examined since meati clogged with wax, or bulging or scarred eardrums are readily seen and remedied. Although these, if present, may not significantly contribute to poor auditory attention, they certainly do not help and are an obstacle easily removed. The problem is always that although intact eyes and ears may mean that a child hears and sees, it does not mean with these children that they look or listen. Whether they in fact do so is extremely difficult to judge from their behaviour. There are various steps which can be taken in order to elicit visual and auditory response. These are described below, but should they be of no avail after e.g. 6 months, and there is no evidence of overt pathology in the eye or ear then the recording techniques, such as VER and cochleography, should be considered.

Eliciting some response to sights and sounds may be most unrewarding with such handicapped children but certainly every effort should be made, particularly with their vision, to capture and sustain the child's interest. Faced with a non-looking child it is customary to try stimulating him with, e.g., bright, noisy toys; with such retarded children this is often of little avail. What seems to be more productive is to concentrate the therapeutic programme on establishing head control, combining this with close face-to-face contact with mother or therapists so that the child, held upright, learns to balance his head at the same time confronted by the visual impression of his mother's face. A simple technique could be used for this. The child is sat facing his mother, on her lap, supported from his head down by a blanket or towel wrapped round him with the ends gathered and held by his mother. By doing this she protracts the child's shoulders, bringing his arms forward so that his hands can touch her face and hair. She can hold closer or farther away but will remain in close physical contact. While moving the towel she can change his position, initially with his head supported, so that he becomes accustomed to a varying position of his head on his trunk. By gradually lowering the towel down the head to the shoulders while moving him in this way she can give him practice in balancing his head, at the same time talking, crooning or singing to him, while he is able to touch her. This close physical contact, combined with emerging head control, has produced visual fixation in a series of seriously handicapped young children within about 6 months. It seems that establishing head control is a necessary preliminary in such children to capturing their visual attention; as if equipping them to hold the world still while in a supported upright position enables them, or incites them, to look.

Once visual interest is obtained, together with the rudiments of head control, the next stage is to progress from this to improving trunk stability in readiness for sitting. There is a simple graduation from handling as described to secure head control; then to lowering the support of the child and changing him from lap to seat so that he can be held while sitting, rotated within a towel or tilted from side to side in play. The aim at this stage is to place the child on a good sitting base with well-abducted hips. This is usually no problem with this type of child, with a seat coming well forward behind the knees and low enough to enable the feet to be flat on the floor. Combined with this handling the child can spend some time in such a seat, partially supported from back and sides, with a tray in front which enables him to bring his arms forward, protracting his shoulders and handling objects bimanually in the mid-line. Since the major concern of treatment for these children is to generate spontaneous activity, frequent periods of sitting practice as described, with progressively less support are only one component of his programme. At the same time the child should be handled in ways which improve his trunk rotation and counteract his tendency to flex. These can both be pursued more actively when the child is able to sit more or less unsupported, but at this stage he will need to

137

be helped while lying. It is regrettable that such children are often left for long periods lying supine on their backs, whereas they benefit from lying prone, e.g. over a wedge, thereby extending hips and knees and bringing their arms forward so that they can handle toys or sand and water. The child should also lie on his side so that similarly his hands can be brought forward in front of him, within his visual field, in the hope that he will handle materials placed close to him or his own face. Every effort should be made to encourage this. At the same time his period on the mat should be punctuated by being playfully rolled about and handled; this will not only encourage his trunk rotation but liven him up generally, raise his tone and give him much-needed experience of movement.

When the child has been handled in this way he will perhaps over 2 or 3 years have a much more confident sitting posture and may be well on the way to unsupported sitting. The aim at this stage is to equip the child to sit with sufficient stability and protective responses to enable him to let go and release his hands confidently for work and play. At this stage one emphasis of his programme will be ón table play: handling, reaching and grasping. Two other components can be added to this programme which may be help-ful.

One is to ensure that much of his interest, reaching and playing, is elicited from the side. This is in contrast to a play programme to help a cerebral palsy child who needs to be approached in play from in front so that by engaging in mid-line activities he minimizes the reflex distortions of his movement. A severely retarded child, however, has no such problems and can turn or lean without rendering himself liable to reflex responses. Stimulation from the side in this way is valuable for him because it gives him practice in trunk rotation which he will need to mobilize himself efficiently from a sitting position. Many seriously retarded children, although able to sit efficiently at the age of 5 or 6 years, have the greatest difficulty in raising themselves to their feet because with poor trunk rotation they try to do so by pulling themselves straight up – which is enormously hard work. To be able, and accustomed, to pivot from a sitting position equips such a child more readily to mobilize himself and to stand up.

A second component of his programme at this stage is to en-courage him to weight-bear; that is to extend his hips and knees from a sitting position. Although the 'natural' way to do this is to hold the child's hands from in front and allow him to pull himself up, this only exaggerates flexion because he tends to hang on to the offered hands. What he needs is encouragement to bring his trunk over his centre of gravity; this means that he should lift his hips forward over feet placed firmly on the floor. Positions of the feet are very important at this stage; they need to be plantar-grade (orthopaedic help may be needed here), and should be placed at about his shoulders' width apart. It helps if early efforts are in bare feet so that the child can maximize through his feet the sensory input that the change of posture demands. If the child is lifted at the hips, preferably from behind so that he moves his weight over his feet and is gently urged upwards, he will readily extend at the knees and hips. It may be that a familiar person needs to be in front of him, or the whole activity could be carried out before a mirror to give him confidence. Certainly a great deal of approval should be shown at the moment when he does extend, and bears weight. It is interesting that many seriously handicapped children of this type can be thus persuaded to bear their weight from either a sitting or a supported crouch position, whereas if they are lifted up for this purpose in the same way as a normal toddler, i.e. from holding them under the arms, they will simply flex their knees and hips and leave the parent or therapist holding them in the air.

The final stages of a programme for such a child are to give him practice in raising and lowering himself from sitting or crouching; to improve sitting balance and use of his hands; and by helping him enjoy rolling and trunk rotation to aim at rolling into sitting, and from sitting to rotate into supported standing with patient encouragement. Some of these children mobilize themselves very efficiently by flexing their hips and draw their knees underneath them when lying prone, then thrusting up into high kneeling they stand up from that position. However it is not uncommon to find these children resistive to prone-lying so that they may not tolerate it long enough to practise or enjoy movement play of this sort.

Once weight-bearing, with reasonable trunk rotation, the child is able, at least with support, to stand up from a chair or lavatory or bed, and to sit back on them again. Repeated practice at this in his daily life, and a varied play programme of movement experience, will give him enough motor capability to launch out with a few steps

Table 9.3 Outline of treatment programme for reducing motor handicap in retarded group

Aim: A listening, looking child with head control and visually directed movements; with stable sitting and hands released and available for play and self-help; with capacity to weight-bear and avoid needing to be lifted and carried; perhaps eventually to walk

Sitting, table play	Handling, mat play
1. Stabilizing head control; visual interest	Throughout Ensure changes in position; not left in supine lying
2. Improve trunk stability, good sitting base, seat support to back of knees, well abducted hips, feet flat on floor	Rolling, toys etc. placed to side. Lie alongside to 'talk'
3. Improve trunk control and protective responses. Rocking in semi-supported sitting	Prone lying over wedge. Encourage use of hands, lie on a raised surface to obtain face-to-face stimulation
4. Unsupported sitting: release hands for tactile play, aim at visually directed reaching etc., hand feeding	
5. Encourage trunk rotation approach from side	Flex hips in prone to encourage crouch and thence extend into kneeling or squat sitting
6. Encourage weight-bearing from sitting, turning in supported standing. Raising and lowering trunk. Extend trunk over hips, ensure plantar-grade feet	Games involving falling from sitting to lying to help confidence and balancing reaction
7. With stabilized standing, encourage forward movement	

himself. Whether he does so or not then depends mainly on the confidence inspired by parents or staff, or the ingenuity shown in exciting him to move in this unaccustomed way. However the major purposes of this programme, which may well take at least 5 or 6 years, are to enable a helpless disinterested child to be capable of weight-bearing so that he will not have to be lifted when older and heavier; to achieve stable sitting with hands released to push a wheelchair; to feed himself; to help dress and perhaps to signal his needs; and to balance sufficiently to sit on the lavatory or to stand with support.

TREATMENT PROGRAMMES FOR CEREBRAL PALSIED GROUP

Cerebral palsy in a mentally handicapped child results commonly from a deficiency in the blood supply to the brain. This can happen at different times, though usually within the perinatal period, affecting different parts of the brain to varying degrees. There is therefore an array of diverse motor handicaps which can occur in combination and with varying severity, so that it is difficult to outline a programme sequence applicable to all these children (Finnie, 1971). There are three common forms of motor disability: spasticity, the result of damage to the motor cortex and corticospinal pathways; ataxia produced by cerebellar damage; and athetosis following damage to the basal ganglia and extrapyramidal pathways. Each of these handicaps is significantly different from the others so a number of basic principles can be suggested to apply to each in turn.

The Spastic Child

The basic difficulty of the spastic child is that his tone increases sharply when he moves, and he has little control in directing his movement because it is very easily distorted by reflex patterns which may be released by the position of his head or trunk and by the level of excitation in his brain. He is a child, therefore, who is particularly vulnerable to posture and head position, to the level of arousal at which he works and plays, and to the direction of any movement to the side since the stiffening spasm and reflex distortion of his efforts is worse if these involve turning his head. It follows that his motor programme, although in detail it needs specialized physiotherapy and teaching, has certain basic requirements. In contrast to the retarded child the spastic needs to be handled in a way which helps him to grade his arousal and movements; his environment should be calm, his handling consistent and predictable; parents and staff should always herald their

141

approach so that he is not startled and should play or work with him in a way which is explained, regular and therefore easily anticipated. Best results are obtained if great care is taken to support his trunk; to assist his head control so that the child is not constantly vulnerable to spasms induced by the need to check and counteract any change in balance or posture. The child needs a stable sitting situation to release his hands; indeed, even to be really aware of his hands. Play or work with his hands is usually easiest for him in the mid-line, if possible using both hands together, so efforts should be made to provide him with such activities which also supinate his wrist and open his fingers. As much practice as possible of grip release, and grading the power of his grip, is helpful. A good deal of work will be needed to reduce adductor spasm of his hips which will pull his legs together both in sitting and in supported standing, thus narrowing his sitting base and making him feel more unstable. Exercises increasing hip adduction and extension are valuable, as are seats with a central pommel with the same well-fitting characteristics as described for the retarded child.

These children should have regular hip X-rays, and a careful watch should be kept on how stiff in flexion and adduction these joints are. They are vulnerable to dislocation and a regular orthopaedic consultation is imperative for their proper management. Since the major aim for the retarded spastic is a good sitting position with reasonable hand-use, well-abducted hips with a minimum of flexion deformity is very important. It may well be that sensible handling and physiotherapy will not counteract this adequately and the child may need surgical treatment such as adductor tenotomy or anterior obdurator neurectomy. The spasm can be reduced in some cases with diazepam (Valium) or baclofen (Lioresal) (Jukes, 1978) though the former has with some children hypotensive or sedating effect whilst the latter, although promising, is, as yet, in its early stages of use.

The Ataxic Child

Whereas the spastic child is one who has high resting tone and stiffens, often into reflex patterns, when he attempts to move, the ataxic child is floppy with a basic inability to balance. He is reluctant to bear weight, has poor trunk control, reaches with a marked tremor and is often a frightened, hesitant child. The spastic child is frustrated because his movements are dominated and misdirected, whereas the ataxic child is primarily apprehensive, afraid to stand up and terrified at movement when upright. He can best be helped quite simply by respecting his need for reassurances. He should, when required to extend into a weight-bearing situation, be helped by parent or therapist kneeling or crouching at his level so that in the upright position he is face to face with his helper. He should be coaxed to come a short distance towards the helper, and never compelled to walk or face away from her. As he moves forward his path should initially be in a straight line with readily available and visible supports to hand. He should not be encouraged to turn or change direction until later. The ground over which he moves should be flat, and he may well be helped by working and playing in bare feet over surfaces of different textures. Together with these simple tips to encourage his practice in weight-bearing and move-ment he can be helped by more vigorous activity, rolling, tumbling over mats and rolls, in a softened environment so that for him falling or rolling becomes less distressing. He will, as with a spastic child, be helped in manual activities by concentrating on mid-line work and bimanual handling of large toys like piling blocks. Some ataxic children, even quite severely affected and mentally retard-ed, become mobile though stumbling and accident prone, whereas others remain unable or unprepared to bear weight unsupported. It does seem that a crucial factor in success or failure is the child's confidence. Although obviously related to the severity of their ataxia and their retardation some children, more successfully reassured than others, are prepared to try moving and standing. Cultivating this confidence should be the mainstay of any treat-ment programme.

The Athetoid Child

The spastic child stiffens and becomes frustrated; the ataxic child stumbles and becomes afraid; but the athetoid child is the jerking wriggler. Defects in the basal ganglia extrapyramidal system pre-vent the child from any efficient grading of muscle action around a joint, interfering with aim and inducing involuntary movements of a writhing and jerking nature. Just as a spastic child stiffens with

143

effort, the athetoid jerks or writhes, so that the aim of therapy is similarly to equip him to control these involuntary movements as best he can. As with the spastic child, a first objective is good head control; a stable sitting position with attention to any adductor spasm that may be present is an important preliminary. The same precautions apply as with a spastic child and the same graded sequence from well-supported sitting in a mould or suitable chair can progress to increasing practice with less support. In the same way stability of trunk and head is imperative before the child can put his hands to use. A second objective is to assess his vision and hearing; hearing defects are common and a high proportion of athetoids have gross refractive error of vision. It is of little avail to help a child stabilize his posture in the hope that he will direct his movements efficiently if his attention is difficult to capture and the visual direction of his movements defective. If he is helped to have reasonable visual monitoring and stable posture then a third component of treatment, important from the beginning, is to bring his hands into his visual field. He, too, will be helped by mid-line bimanual activities, piling blocks, lifting hoops, raising and lowering within the mid-line. A fourth factor is the need to help him to execute his movements in as regular and drill-like way as possible, i.e. to enable him to perform tasks as far as possible without directing his attention to the effort he is making and the sequence of movements he must perform. The task confronting the athetoid in his motor learning, as indeed with our own everyday skills utilizing extrapyramidal control such as writing, dressing and shaving, is that they should not be thought about during their execution. The skill built by all of us into the fluent sequence of movements which we use in everyday activities depends on their being automatic, and the tragedy of the athetoid child is that the more 'consciously' he attends to his efforts at establishing a sequence the more difficult its execution becomes. He is best helped, as with other cerebral palsied children, by a calm, confident setting, but with an emphasis on the end-product of a task rather than the sequence of steps to acquire it. The more he can execute these sequences without directing his attention too closely to them the more efficiently he will perform. It is for this reason that the group drill technique of play and motor learning used in conductive education is so successful. Athetoid children make greatest progress by acquiring in a regular repetitive way a simple sequence of acts which are so constructed that the body performs in the mid-line; e.g. lifting both hands to the back of the chair to raise themselves, each step becoming as automatic as possible through repetition, joining in with a group of similarly instructed children. Through this mechanism Peto methods have achieved considerable success with this type of disability.

Table 9.4 Outline of programmes for reducing motor handicap in cerebral palsy group

These are broad principles; the expertise of therapists and teachers is needed to formulate individual programmes

Spastic (stiff)	Ataxic (unsteady)	Athetoid (involuntary movement)
High tone, tendency to spasm. Reflex distortion of movement particularly if excited or agitated	Low tone; cannot balance. Tremor. Stumbling. Frightened	Involuntary jerking. Writhing, misdirected movements. Much worse if agitated
Aim: grade arousal and strength of movement	Aim: reassure, practise, harness compensatory controls	Aim: 'automatic' simple sequences of movement
Stabilize head control, and trunk with gradually reduced support. Often helped by counteracting extensor spasm in sitting.	Gradual practice in confident atmosphere to weight-bear, step, turn. Helped with 'falling' practice in soft surroundings	Regular repetitive 'sequenced' movements. Stable head control. Helped by emphasis on bimanual mid-line play and tasks

AIDS AND EQUIPMENT

There are a variety of aids which can be used to assist parents and staff in their efforts to improve the motor efficiency of cerebral palsied and retarded children. In the early stages the main emphasis is on handling and postural support which would be primarily within the arms of parents and staff. Later a well-constructed postural mould and good supportive chairs are important. The aim is to provide support in appropriate posture without too much restriction, if possible combining these with a means of reducing such support progressively (e.g. chairs with lower backs). For work aimed at movement experience and balance, rolls are important;

they can be sat across to help abduction, kneeled or rolled over to assist crouching, high kneeling and protective arm extension. Large inflated balls can be used similarly with the additional advantage of allowing a low-toned child lying across it to be bounced onto his feet. Firm wedges assist prone lying and should be of varying sizes and heights, so that the child's length of trunk and the freeing of his arms can be accommodated. In some cases walking frames, e.g. lobster-pot aids, are valuable in the child with reasonable trunk control but little motivation for moving; these enable him with comparatively little effort to gain a change of scene under his own steam. All supports to help weight-bearing are valuable; for instance standing-frames and inset tables. A table or flat surface in front of a child should always be regarded as a platform for toys or anything to feel or grab; it is useful to have a raised containing rim, or objects tied to the table top, so that they can be retrieved by the child himself.

Aids for self-help will rely mainly on the common sense and experience of staff. Balancing on the lavatory will depend not only on sitting posture and trunk control but also on the design of the lavatory itself; or supports around it. In this as with much equipment a good model is not necessarily expensive, if designed by involved staff (Lyle, 1978). (Assistance in this respect can be obtained from the Aids and Equipment Department, Spastics Society, 16 Fitzroy Square, London, W1.) Similarly with feeding; sitting stability is important, as is an appropriate chair and a table sufficiently high and close to minimize, at least initially, the distance a child needs to move his hand from plate to mouth. A whole array of additional aids for feeding include fixed plates with a built-up end to facilitate loading the spoon, thickened spoon and fork handles set at various angles, and two-handled cups with a lid to prevent spilling. Clothing of such children, if they are to be helped to cope with dressing themselves, must be simple in design, fairly loose and comfortable, with a minimum of zips and buttons. The pull-on–off shirts and jerseys are useful as are poncho/cape-style rainproofs and coats which can be slipped on quickly, with the child in his chair, and equally easily removed. Footwear is often a source of some anxiety and orthopaedic opinion is valuable, but in general wearing well-fitting footwear with some work and play in bare feet is usually adequate.

Details of toys for handicapped children are discussed elsewhere in this volume, but for the motor handicapped it is helpful to concentrate on those toys which can be enjoyed with minimum manipulation. Since many of these children have sensory defects and problems of body image, small mirrors, vibrating or whirring toys, or toys which light up can help the child direct his attention. Care should be taken that the toys should be, if not unbreakable, at least splinterproof, and should be easily cleaned. It is always of great value if any toy which 'works' can be set going or stopped by the child himself.

MANAGEMENT AS A TEAM EFFORT

Contribution of various therapists to remedial programmes for this group of children will inevitably depend on the availability, enthusiasm and expertise of the therapists involved. They can be of immense value but there are two ways in which they can be misused. The first is that they can be under-used; accepting that they are in short supply their help may not be sought because motor handicapped, severely retarded children are too often felt to be incapable of benefiting. The second is that an individual therapist may be confronted with a child and expected to take sole responsibility for his programme without the opportunity of discussing it with doctors, other therapists, teachers and parents, so that the total needs of the child are lost. The therapist alone may feel responsible for securing a particular skill; e.g. instructions may be given to her to develop a 'feeding programme' with no steps taken to ensure that her advice is carried through to all mealtimes. Effective therapy for these children does not consist of treatment sessions but of a lifestyle which, to carry it through the day, needs the co-ordinated involvement as a team of all those who handle, talk, teach, and play with him. The role adopted by each member of this team will vary with their personal background, the time available to them, the extent they feel involved together, and the way the child responds to each of them, as well as their participation in the sort of programme outlined above. In these programmes aimed at reducing motor handicap the contribution of parents, physio- and play therapists and teachers will be self-evident, since they, as far as they are available, are directly involved with handling and stimulating the child. They should, above all, work together. Some arrangement which ensures a consistent agreed management and respects the child's own response is essential.

Using intelligible speech is such a crowning achievement for these children, so rewarding to parents and staff alike that the speech therapist often finds herself under quite unrealistic pressure to 'get the child to talk'. Too few of us are as aware as she is of the complexity of skills needed simply to articulate coherently, let alone put a few words together in a useful phrase. So her expertise can be of great value in adjusting the perspective of the team in a communication programme. She will demonstrate ways to help the child listen to speech. She will emphasize the need to appreciate and encourage the simplest vocal utterances, responding to the inflection and cadence of his voice and to his facial expression. Over and above these aids she will, together with psychologist colleagues, advise on the way language which the child hears can be structured and regularized. Her expertise in all forms of oral movement and, of particular importance, sensitivity should be harnessed to help in feeding programmes as well as improving articulation (Treharne, 1979).

The main value of music therapy (Alvin, 1972) is the pleasure it affords, but in addition it has three practical assets for such children. It can help focus their auditory attention and give practice not only in listening but in discriminating important pitch changes and sound qualities like fast and slow rhythms. It can be used to encourage vocalization with, e.g., playing an instrument (which in its turn can improve mouth sensitivity) particularly if the child is able to vocalize into a microphone with a feedback device so that he can hear his own voice. Since most children enjoy making music, however simply, it can also encourage spontaneous motor activity, and refine control of movements; children may more readily improve their arm movement banging a drum than with more formal physiotherapy, and can learn to control these movements by, e.g., stopping and starting with the music or with changes in its rhythm. Art therapy similarly is of great value in enabling the child to enjoy some simple creative act of his own; with finger-paints he can produce his own 'picture' with the simplest and most restricted of movements. With approval of his efforts, and applause for his own picture, he can be coaxed into more flexible directed move-

148

ment such as round and round scribble or dabbing dots. In all these activities, with the child's enjoyment comes incentive to gain and maintain better posture so that he can achieve better hand-control. This in turn encourages visual monitoring of his movements, allows him some choice of expression of his feelings and gives him a sense of creating something of his own.

The importance of the psychologist's contribution to assessment and formulating education/training programmes for the handicapped is self-evident throughout the book, where full justice of it will have been done by its practitioners. With motor handicaps the insight psychologists provide into perceptual difficulties or unsuspected assets can be particularly valuable, as can their expertise in breaking down tasks into a learning sequence. The order in which these sequences are tackled, and the manner in which each step is secured, is rarely as simple as it seems, so the psychologist may well be a central figure in working out the details of any programme (Beresford and Casey, 1978; Kiernan *et al.*, 1978). It must be emphasized however that motor handicapped retarded children need help not only in learning skills but also in executing them. Priority must always be given to overcoming the obstacles and frustrations this imposes.

If he is effectively to guide the team, the doctor must assess the child's needs and how they are to be met. This should mean a lot more than defining the handicap and co-ordinating the work of others. He must also be able to evaluate the child's disability in explaining how it interferes with his functioning, to recognize the need for and secure (or avoid) further investigations necessary to clarify this, and to understand what the results of those investigations imply. He must present these findings as a coherent picture to the team, and especially to the child's parents. Together they can then agree on a series of objectives but may well need to establish priorities among them. It is the doctor's responsibility to advise on such priorities, on how long each part of the programme may take, what is likely to go wrong, and how to anticipate and safeguard against it. As the work of the team proceeds he must appreciate the limits of the programme yet maintain enthusiasm. He must keep treatment aims clear yet ensure that all those involved see the patient as a person and not simply a challenge to their own particular clinical expertise. By recurrently taking stock he must keep the team working together with unified and agreed purpose seen by all, particularly parents, to be for the child's benefit.

References

Cunningham, C. and Sloper, P. (1978). *Helping your Handicapped Baby.* (London: Souvenir Press)

Scott, J. (1979). Stimulating Stanley – one small step at a time. Nursing care study. *Nursing Mirror,* 11 January, p. 34

Finnie, N. (1971). *Handling the Young Cerebral Palsied at Home.* (London: Heineman)

Jukes, M. A. (ed.) (1978). *Baclofen: Spasticity and Cerebral Pathology.* (Northampton: Cambridge Medical Publications)

Lyle, W. J. (1978). Do-it-yourself toilet training aid. *Spastics News,* July

Treharne, D. (1979). Management of feeding difficulties. *Nursing Times,* **75,** 108

Alvin, J. (1972). Music for the Handicapped Child. *The Cerebral Palsied Child.* (London: Oxford University Press)

Jeavons, T. (1975). *Multihandicap and Art.* Meldreth Manor School Occasional Papers. (The Spastics Society)

Beresford, A. and Casey, W. (1978). A simple mobility programme for profoundly handicapped adults. *Apex,* **6,** 19

Kiernan, C., Jordan, R. and Saunders, C. (1978). Human Horizon Series. (London: Souvenir Press)

10

COMMUNICATION

M. Walker

The White Paper of 1971 reported a survey of severely mentally handicapped adults in hospitals for the mentally handicapped in Wessex which stated that one in three had speech defects. The latest report (1979) of the Development Team for the Mentally Handicapped states that on the basis of reports by staff in hospitals for the mentally handicapped, 57% of children and 22% of adults suffer from speech defects.

It is therefore of the greatest importance to assess the type of communication, if any, used *by* and *to* a mentally handicapped person, in order to judge if it is adequate and in keeping with his/her general level of ability and degree of handicap. If it is not, and frequently this is the case, then treatment should be given so that some form of communication, however basic it may be, can be established.

Until this is done, all management, training and development of the mentally handicapped child/adult will be hampered. Furthermore, the lack of communication may (and frequently does) influence behaviour to such an extent that assessment in any sphere becomes extremely difficult and often impossible.

The Role of the Speech Therapist in Mental Handicap

Everyone involved with the mentally handicapped should share in the responsibility of establishing effective communication. Having said that though, not everyone is equally trained and equipped to initiate and carry out programmes without assistance.

Undoubtedly, the speech therapist is the expert. Her training equips her to assess and treat problems affecting the delay in, the lack, and breakdown of communication over the entire IQ range from the cradle to the grave. No other profession has this unique therapeutic experience and training, or indeed such a broad overview.

Sadly, speech therapists are in short supply, often having only limited sessions in an establishment, or often there is no provision at all. With this in mind, this chapter is written by a speech therapist, in an attempt not to replace speech therapists, but to make the contribution of those who are available more effective by sharing knowledge and offering direction so that the communication needs of the mentally handicapped can be more adequately met. It is hoped that the information and suggestions here will ensure greater participation and confidence in others working with, and caring for, the mentally handicapped.

COMMUNICATION AND THE MENTALLY HANDICAPPED

In the normal child communication develops in well-defined progressive stages. For example (all ages are approximate):

From 6 weeks to 6 months	Child experiments making sounds for pleasure (babbling).
From 6 months to 9 months	Vocalizes and gestures to gain attention.
From 9 months to 12 months	Understands few familiar words like 'no', 'bye-bye'; knows own name, shouts to attract attention.
12 months	Responds to own name, understands simple instructions if accompanied by gesture, often speaks first words.

15 months	Says two to six recognizable words.
18 months	Says six to twenty recognizable words.
2 years	Uses fifty recognizable words, understands many more, begins to link words in two-word phrases.

For further details of subsequent stages, see Developmental Progress Scales (Sheridan) in Information Section.

If communication develops in the mentally handicapped, similar progressive stages can be identified, but they occur at a very much later age and the progress from one stage to another is very much slower.

How far communication will develop and whether it develops at all will depend largely on the severity of the individual's handicap, combined with how much or how little opportunity there has been for them to receive the correct stimulation and training to encourage communication to develop.

Communication should be considered in its broadest sense, so that it covers speech, natural gesture, signing, the use of symbols and even body language.

It is also very important that it is seen as a two-way process comprising:

> *the person transmitting the message,* and
> *the person receiving it.*

These two aspects of communication are equally important. All too often a mentally handicapped person's ability to communicate is assessed in detail but the other aspect – the speech of those caring, living and working with the child/adult in his/her environment – is overlooked. Ideally both should communicate at the same level for it to be effective.

In order to judge if the two-way process is satisfactory, the following procedure is recommended.

GENERAL PROCEDURE FOR ESTABLISHING EFFECTIVE COMMUNICATION

1) Assessment

A careful assessment of the type of communication and of the factors influencing it should be made of:

(a) the mentally handicapped person; and
(b) the people in that person's environment

2) Evaluation

The results of the assessment should then be evaluated and this should indicate if treatment is necessary or not.

3) Treatment

If treatment is required then treatment procedures should be designed and put into practice. These should be:

(a) suitable for the child/adult's needs as shown in the assessment;
(b) workable within the child/adult's environment by those staff/parents who have to carry them out.

Now let us look at each of these areas in more detail.

1. ASSESSMENT

Assessments should therefore be aimed at pinpointing the stage of development which the mentally handicapped person has reached in order to be able:

(a) to gauge one's own communication, whether it be speech, signing or symbols, to suit their level of understanding;
(b) to compare their level of communication with their general level of ability, to see if it matches;
(c) to plan a treatment programme which starts at their current level and takes them from that stage to the next and so on.

To find the starting point the child/adult's level should be assessed on each of the following components of communication.

(a) *Comprehension of Language* (how much of our communica- do they understand?);

(b) *Expressive Language* (how do they express themselves?);
(c) *Production of Communication* (can they produce, e.g. actual speech sounds, movement for signing?);
(d) *Additional Handicaps* (e.g. hearing loss, cleft palate, physical handicap, etc?);
(e) *Motivation and General Behaviour* (e.g. poor concentration, hyperactivity, etc.).

COMPREHENSION OF LANGUAGE

What do we want to know about Comprehension of Language?

a) The Mentally Handicapped Child/Adult

How much do the children/adults understand of what we say?

If they understand little of our speech, are they simply responding to facial expression, gestures and situational clues? For example, if everyone is putting their coats on to go outside, the child may realize that he is to go out also: not because of the spoken instruction but because of the obvious clues around him.

Can they generalize a concept they have learned? For example do they realize that a 'chair' is not just the one they sit on but refers to all designs and types of chairs in differing environments?

How limited is their understanding of our vocabulary?

How limited is their memory for retention of speech?

What is their level of attention?

Does the child have a hearing loss? If so, this will affect understanding of our speech.

b) The Child/Adult's Environment

Is the level of the spoken language that we use within the range of their understanding?

Do we use vocabulary that they have had experience of, and can understand?

Does our level of communication, whether by simple speech, sign or symbols, match their simple level of understanding?

Do we adjust the length of what we say or sign to match their memory capacity?

Do we make sure we have their attention before we start communicating and adjust the length of what we say to match their

155

attention-span? For example, with someone with very short attention-span it is better to break long instructions into two parts rather than say it in one long sentence, e.g. 'pick up the cup' (wait until they do it), then 'put it on the table' instead of: 'pick up the cup and put it on the table'.

EXPRESSIVE LANGUAGE

What do we want to know about Expressive Language?

a) The Mentally Handicapped Child/Adult

How does the child/adult express himself, e.g. grunts/sounds, gestures/signs, single words, phrases, sentences?

How does he/she make his needs known?

Does he create his own expressive speech/gestures, however crudely, or simply imitate or repeat words or whole phrases he has learnt without understanding? This can often be misleading, they may talk a lot and it may seem relevant; therefore check to see if adult/child understands what he/she is saying.

How limited is expressive vocabulary?

Does the child have a hearing loss? If so they will have difficulty in monitoring their own and our speech.

b) The Child/Adult's Environment

Do we notice and encourage forms of communication other than speech, no matter how primitive?

Do we utilize the above, as a baseline on which to build communication?

Do we provide training in alternative means of communication as well as speech, to provide additional medium for communication, e.g. signing or symbol system?

Do we provide clear examples of expressive speech at an appropriate level for their ability for them to experience and learn from?

Method of Assessment

Assessment of comprehension of language and expressive language

Both of these may be assessed on formal language assessments such as Reynell Developmental Language Scales, ITPA, Carrow, etc. or informally on developmental checklists such as Gunzburg's Progressive Assessment Charts, IMS/BIMH checklist.

The formal assessments are the most satisfactory form of assessment and wherever possible should be given. They can only be administered by speech therapists, psychologists, teachers and others who have attended a specific course on the administration and evaluation of the test. The results provide a language level and indicate where further specific assessment is required, to investigate other associated problem areas, e.g. dysphasia, dyspraxia. Often a combination of assessments is required to provide all the necessary information.

Development checklists can be used by anyone with sufficient professional understanding. Generally they present basic skills such as communication, social skills, movement, play and self-help as schedules of developmental sequences against which the individual's level of attainment can be noted. The amount of details given in the sequential stages differs from one checklist to another. They provide a general and useful indication of development and a comparison of one skill with another. Frequently language-stimulation programmes are associated with the checklist.

Assessment of Vocabulary

This can be measured on formal assessments such as Peabody Vocabulary Test and the English Picture Vocabulary Test, if the intellectual level of the individual is within the range of the test. They are available to speech therapists and teachers.

Often the handicapped person's experience is very restricted, and test results give little information. It is then necessary to record vocabulary in real-life situations and to relate findings to a developmental vocabulary such as the Makaton Vocabulary.

Assessment of Attention

Reference to the work of Cooper, Moodley and Reynell (see section on Information) is useful, in order to be able to obtain attention levels.

Assessment of Memory Length for Speech

Memory length is related to general intellectual ability and the capacity generally increases with maturation. The length (signed or spoken) that a person can understand and can express will depend on memory length. Careful observation is required to measure it.

PRODUCTION OF COMMUNICATION

What do we want to know about Production of Communication?

a) The Mentally Handicapped Child/Adult

Is the child/adult physically handicapped? If so how severely does this affect speech and voice production and general movement?

Are there specific speech production problems, e.g. *dysarthria* (neurological damage affecting the speech muscles and causing drooling, swallowing difficulties, clumsy tongue and lip movement and slurred speech) or *articulatory dyspraxia* (neurological damage affecting the learning of speech patterns needed to produce speech sounds)?

Does the child have cleft palate, lip or both?

Is articulation of the actual speech sounds defective or immature, making it difficult to understand what the child is saying?

Has the child a hearing loss? This will also affect intelligibility of sound production.

Is voice produced normally and is vocal quality normal?

Are feeding patterns normal? It is important to establish correct patterns as speech sounds develop from these.

Are breathing patterns normal?

b) The Child/Adult's Environment

Do we produce clear articulated speech, so that the child/adult has a good model to copy?

If physical movement is severely restricted are artificial aids offered, e.g. mechanical communication aids, communication board, symbol system?

Method of Assessment – Production of Communication

Problems such as dyspraxia and dysarthria, may be associated with other physical handicaps or may occur in isolation. They will require specialized assessment by a speech therapist.

Poor or Defective Articulation

This may be linked with physical handicap, or may occur on its own, and frequently does. It is often related in the mentally handicapped to immaturity or to poor muscle tone and sometimes to the disproportion of speech organs. Assessment and advice by a speech therapist is necessary.

Feeding Patterns

It is most important to observe and relate these to the child/adult's general level of development.

The sounds used in speech develop from feeding. For example the sounds 'p, b, m, c/k, g' from sucking and swallowing, 't, d, n' develop from teething, and later sounds involving the cheek muscles from chewing. If feeding has been a problem and abnormal patterns persist, then sound production development will be seriously affected. See sections on Information for further details on assessment and management.

Cleft Palate

The assessment of the speech-production problems associated with a cleft of the palate or lip or a submucous cleft needs specialist assessment by a speech therapist.

ADDITIONAL HANDICAPS

What Additional Handicaps are present affecting Development of Communication?

a) The Mentally Handicapped Child/Adult

Is the child/adult known to have a hearing loss?
Are any of these warning signs present?

Does child/adult respond abnormally to loud noises?
Does child/adult watch speaker's face a great deal?
Has child/adult had frequent colds, catarrh?
Has child/adult had frequent doses of antibiotics for infections?
Is there an excessive amount of wax in ears?
If child has Down's (mongolism) syndrome, cleft palate, cerebral palsy, particularly athetosis, check to see if he/she has a high-frequency hearing loss.

Does child/adult have any visual defects?
Are there any perceptual problems? These may be visual or auditory – child/adult may see and hear but has difficulty in perceiving them.
Are there any specific language problems such as: *developmental dysphasia* (a specific neurological problem, child/adult has difficulty in appreciating the meaning of spoken language and in expressing its thoughts in language which is not in proportion to the level of intelligence); *autism* (complex condition, child/adult has difficulty in interpreting and coding incoming stimuli; stereotyped learning occurs from very concrete experience; talks in stereotyped speech patterns if speech develops to that level.)

b) The Child/Adult's Environment

Do we realize the degree of impairment of any additional handicap?
Do we make allowances for this when we communicate?
Do we provide child/adult with training in an additional alternative communication system as well as speech, e.g. a signing or symbol system to provide multisensory input?

METHOD OF ASSESSMENT – ADDITIONAL HANDICAPS

Assessment of Hearing Loss

If a child/adult is suspected of having a hearing loss then he/she should be referred through the family doctor or school medical officer, for specialist assessment, to an ENT consultant or specialist audiologist. An experienced audiometrician working with the specialist, who has expertise in the management of mentally handicapped people in a test situation, will be able to select an appropriate method of assessment to suit the child/adult. Routine screening procedures to test hearing are generally *not* adequate for the mentally handicapped person.

Assessment of Visual Defects

The child/adult with a visual defect requires specialist assessment and should be referred through his doctor or school medical officer to the ophthalmologist and the orthoptist when necessary.

Specific Language Problems, e.g. Dysphasia, Autism

The child with either of these requires specialized assessment by a speech therapist.

Perceptual Problems

These may affect vision or hearing and again require specialized assessment by an experienced professional person.

MOTIVATION AND GENERAL BEHAVIOUR

What Do We want to Know about Motivation and General Behaviour?

a) The Mentally Handicapped Child/Adult

Is child/adult interested and motivated to communicate?
Does he/she relate to people in his/her environment?
Does child have behaviour problems?
Is the child/adult's behaviour disruptive?
Does child/adult try to manipulate the people in the environment?
Does the child play at all, or show any signs of simple play?

b) The Child/Adult's Environment

Do we encourage and reward his/her attempts to communicate enough?

Does the environment provide experience in communication and is it at the appropriate level?

Is the environment relaxed, happy and sympathetic?

Are there opportunities in the environment to encourage and teach the mentally handicapped how to play?

Method of Assessment

Assessment of Motivation and General Behaviour

These can be assessed by careful observation and on checklists such as Gunzburg's Progressive Assessment Charts or one of the others referred to in the chapter on the Behaviour approach.

Assessment of Play

This may be assessed on a formal assessment (Lowe and Costello) if child/adult comes within age range of test. Otherwise observe and look for any signs of early play, described on developmental scales such as Sheridan, 1975; Jeffree and McConkey, 1976.

2. EVALUATION

Hopefully by now, after carrying out the assessment, it should be possible to describe the handicapped person's communicative ability for each of the components of communication, i.e. comprehension of language, expressive language, production of communication, additional handicaps, motivation and general behaviour.

Do not be concerned if this information is sparse and tends to be negative. If a handicapped person's skill in communication is extremely limited or simply does not exist at all, then it cannot be assessed more favourably. At least by assessing it, confirmation of the severity of the handicap has been gained.

Having gathered all this information, what does one do with it and how does one evaluate it, in order to judge if treatment is needed or not?

Suggested Procedure

1. Find out the overall level of ability of the person. Look at the ability in its broadest sense, e.g. obtain a level for self-help

skills: dressing, feeding, toileting, occupation/work if any. Refer to psychological assessments if available for further information and to confirm general intellectual level of ability and level of basic skills. Also observe the individual yourself. Quite often, there is an inconsistent pattern, with some skills being better developed than others, but generally an average level of ability for that individual will emerge and this is what is required.

If you are not certain of the developmental levels of ability then consult development tables or charts (see section on Information). It is often a good idea to do this even if one has had considerable experience of normal child development, since it is often difficult to recall the exact developmental sub-stage or to remember how this related to other areas of development.

2. When one has a knowledge of the overall level of ability of the handicapped person then estimate:
   (a) the type of communication that a handicapped person with that level of ability should have;
   (b) the type of communication that people in contact with them should use.

3. Compare the *actual* levels of the handicapped person's communication, i.e. the results of the assessment described earlier, under comprehension of language, expressive language, etc. with the *expected* levels of communication estimated in point (2) above. Ideally both should be the same.

   As a rough guide one would expect, if communication is satisfactory, that comprehension of language approximately equates to the overall level of ability. Expressive language will be the same as or just below the level of comprehension of language, by about 3–6 months. Attention-span, memory retention for speech and the production of communication should be the same as the individual's overall level of ability.

4. If the 'actual' and the 'expected' levels of communication are the same or almost the same then this indicates that the person's communication is adequate. Specific treatment will not be required but continued opportunities to use and receive

plenty of stimulating communication will be essential so that the current level of functioning can be maintained and possibly increased.

If the 'actual' and 'expected' levels are not the same, then identify where the differences lie, by carefully comparing the detailed results previously obtained for communication with the expected levels for the various components of communication. Identify where the discrepancy occurs. For example, does the discrepancy occur in comprehension of language, or in the production of speech sounds? Also note the extent of the discrepancy, e.g. how delayed is this component of communication compared with the expected level.

Try to account for the difference. Look for obvious additional handicaps which could affect development specifically in communication e.g. hearing loss; cleft palate, poor and inappropriate stimulation, etc.

5. Finally, summarize clearly the components of communication requiring action and treatment.

3. TREATMENT

Assuming that the assessment and evaluation has been comprehensive and that action such as referral for any necessary, specific examinations has been done, e.g. tests for hearing and vision, then turn your attention to treatment.

Approach treatment in a very 'down-to-earth', practical manner, bearing in mind two essential points, mentioned earlier, that treatment plans should be designed to be:

(a) suitable for the child/adult's needs as shown in the assessment; and

(b) workable within the child/adult's environment by those staff/parents who have to carry them out.

There are several comprehensive treatment/remedial programmes available now, e.g. Portage, Distar, which include communication programmes within a total programme of stimulation. There are also specific language schemes, e.g. the Derbyshire Language Scheme, the Peabody Language Development Kit. Finally, there are the alternative systems of communication which may be taught, e.g. The Makaton Vocabulary, The Paget-Gorman Sign System and Bliss. (The Makaton Vocabulary is not only an alternative means of communication but also a structured language scheme.)

Any one of these methods may be used on its own, or as has been shown in practice they can be used in combination, e.g. Portage/Makaton; Bliss/Makaton; Bliss/Paget-Gorman Sign System: Derbyshire Language Scheme/Makaton. Alternatively treatment programmes may be devised to meet individual needs by a suitably qualified person, which may not involve any of these 'package type' schemes and be equally effective. The deciding factor in making the choice must be the two points (a) and (b) mentioned earlier.

It is often difficult to know which choice to make, especially if the people having to make the decision do not have the professional experience to enable them to confidently assess the merits of the various methods available and to relate them to the needs of the individual. For example, adult training centre, hostel or hospital staff who feel a programme to be necessary, should seek the advice of a speech therapist. If your establishment does not have a regular speech therapy service then contact the area speech therapy service at the area health authority to enquire if a speech therapist could visit to advise. The speech therapist should be able to advise on the choice of an appropriate method, provide an initial demonstration of the techniques and suggest a method of monitoring progress, even if he/she cannot carry out the actual treatment.

If an individual is attending a school or other department at which a programme is in operation then it should become established practice for everyone involved in his/her management and care including parents, to be provided with some instruction so that the programme is carried out, wherever the person may be.

The scope of this chapter unfortunately does not permit discussion of the various therapeutic techniques or the use of equipment. However, references to sources which will provide practical information are given in the sections on Information. In addition to this the following points are offered for consideration in approaching and selecting treatment procedures for the mentally handicapped.

165

CONSIDERATIONS FOR CHOICE OF TYPE OF TREATMENT

1. Consider the specific communication needs of the child/adult, e.g. poor comprehension of language; limited or no expressive speech.
2. Consider any additional handicaps that are present, treatment procedures must be flexible enough to accommodate these further handicaps.
3. Consider behaviour and relate this to choice of programme. It is no good for example choosing a programme involving group work if attention is so low that it demands one-to-one treatment sessions.
4. Consider the environment and decide who will carry out treatment.
5. Discover how much time they can practically provide to give treatment.
6. Consider whether staff providing treatment will be sufficiently skilled and confident to use the treatment procedures efficiently. How easy will it be for them to be provided with instruction and to gain this expertise?
7. Assuming that the treatment has successful results, consider how easy it will be for other staff on the fringe, and parents, to become involved and suitably trained in the treatment procedure, so that they can participate and extend the scheme.

FINAL SUMMARY

Remember, from the outset, that the aims of treatment should be clearly defined and plans carefully structured starting at the current level of capability of the individual and progressing through small developmental stages to increase the communication skill.

Choose appropriate treatment procedures that one has confidence in. It is far better to select a simple scheme with clear, precise and practical aims, that can be carried out easily in a work/home situation, than to undertake a procedure which is too sophisticated and demanding to be applied by non-professionals.

Maintain your interest by attending conferences, seminars, training courses; read current articles and literature on treatment and management and try occasionally to visit centres similar to your own, to exchange ideas and discuss problems. Re-assess programmes periodically (e.g. every 6 months) to measure if improvement is occurring, and keep simple records to monitor your treatment and ensure that it covers all intended areas of communication development. Also inform others in your centre of your results, and be prepared to discuss results and procedures with them.

Make treatment enjoyable, pleasant and meaningful. Remember that communication occurs in every moment of our waking day and that it is not an activity carried out only in set treatment sessions. Be constantly aware of the need to generalize and extend treatment into every 'real life' situation. And, that to begin with, communication can be as simple and spontaneous as an encouraging smile or a reassuring arm around a child's shoulders.

References

Better Services for the Mentally Handicapped (1971). HMSO. Comnd 1683

Development Team for the Mentally Handicapped (2nd Report) (1979)

INFORMATION

Assessments

Formal Assessments to Test Communication and Hearing

Listed below are some of the more widely used tests:

Reynell Development Language Scales (revised) (*age range*: 1½–6 years).
Illinois Test of Psycholinguistic Abilities (*age range*: 2–10 years).
Language Imitation Test (Berry and Mittler) (*age range*: ESN(S) range).
Peabody Picture Vocabulary Test (*age range*: 2½–18 years).
Stycar Hearing Tests (*age range*: 6 months–7 years).
Stycar Language Tests (*age range*: children under 7 years).
All the above are available from NFER Publishing Company

(Test Department), Darville House, 2 Oxford Road East, Windsor, SL4 1DF. Catalogue of tests available giving details and capabilities of each test and the necessary qualifications to administer them.

The Carrow Test for Auditory Comprehension of Language (*age range*: 3–7 years).
    Available from Learning Concepts, 2501 N. Lamar, Austin, Texas 78705, USA.

English Picture Vocabulary Test (Brimar and Dunn).
    Available from Educational Evaluation Enterprises, Owre, Newnham, Gloucestershire.

Developmental Checklist/Development Progress Charts

IMS/BIMH Developmental Checklist (associated with the book *Helping the Retarded*, by Perkins, Capie and Taylor).
    Available from BIMH, Kidderminster.

National Children's Bureau Development Guide and Charts (0–5 years, experimental version).
Handbook and charts available from: National Children's Bureau, 8 Wakley Street, London EC1V 7QE.

PIP Development Charts, by D. Jeffree and R. McConkey.
    Published by Hodder & Stoughton, P.O. Box 702, Mill Road, Dunton Green, Sevenoaks, Kent TN13 2YD.

The Progress Assessment Chart of Social and Personal Development, by H. C. Gunzburg.
    Manual and charts available from: NSMHC Bookshop, 117 Golden Lane, London EC1 0RT.

The REEL Test – Receptive, Expressive Emergent Language Test, by Bzoch and League. (Range 0–3 years)
    Manual available from Henry Kimpton, Publisher and Bookseller, Great Portland Street, London W1. *Comment*: This test is specifically a language test. Stages are small and detailed. Technical jargon is used, therefore the person using it requires a certain amount of specialized understanding. Very useful test.

Formal Assessments to Test Play

Symbolic Play Test (experimental edition), Lowe & Costello (*age range*: 12–36 months).
Available from NFER, Windsor.

Formal Test to Assess Visual Perception

Marianne Frostig Developmental Test of Visual Perception. Available to all Speech Therapists and Teachers (*age range*: 4–8 years; often too advanced for mentally handicapped)
Associated programme available also (*age range*: 3½–7½ years).
Available from NFER, Windsor.

Additional Test Source

The Developmental Potential of Pre-School Children, by Else Haeussermann. (Published by Grune & Stratton.)
Useful reference source of simple informal tests to measure wide variety of developing skills.

Sources of Information on Remedial Approaches and Treatment

Ways and Means. A resource book of aids, methods, materials and systems for use with the language-retarded child. In addition reference is made to Portage, Distar, the Peabody Kits, and other alternative means of communication. Co-ordinator: Trevor Tebbs (Published by Globe Education Ltd., Houndmills, Basingstoke, Hants.)
An excellent resource book covering all current treatment approaches and a review of available equipment and suppliers. Highly recommended.

Material for Language Stimulation. (Published by the College of Speech Therapists, Harold Poster House, 6 Lechmere Road, London NW2 5BU.)
Inexpensive booklet, which provides excellent ideas and suggestions for utilizing familiar remedial equipment as part of a developmental language stimulation programme. Useful in the mental handicap and normal range.

'*Let Me Speak*', by D. Jeffree and R. McConkey.
'*Let Me Play*', by D. Jeffree and R. McConkey.
'*Teaching the Handicapped Child*, by D. Jeffree, R. McConkey and Newton.
(All published by Souvenir Press Ltd; (Human Horizons Series.)

> Excellent sources of practical suggestions for furthering the subject of each book. Primarily designed for parents, but of great value to everyone caring for and working with mentally handicapped. The PIP Development Charts should be used in association with the books (see Developmental Checklist section).

Helping Language Development. A developmental programme for children with early language handicaps, by: Cooper, Moodley and Reynell. (Published by Edward Arnold.)

> Written mainly for speech therapists, psychologists, teachers and medical practitioners. Requires a certain amount of professional understanding. Excellent and effective assessment and stimulation programme. Schedule of attention levels referred to under Assessment references.

Early Language Programme. A programme of activities to aid the development of early language. Compiled by speech therapists and teachers of Education Department of Borough of Kingston. (Published by Royal Borough of Kingston-upon-Thames, Tolworth Tower, Surbiton, Surrey).

> Inexpensive, useful and practical programme to aid the development of language. Devised primarily for the ESN(M) child, but some of the ideas are appropriate for the brighter severely mentally handicapped person.

Helping the Retarded, by Perkins, Taylor and Capie. (Published by British Institute of Mental Handicap, Kidderminster, Worcs.)

> A particularly lucid explanation and illustration of behaviour modification principles. Suggested programmes are given. A very useful developmental checklist is also available.

Helping Mentally Handicapped People in Hospital.

> A report to the Secretary of State for Social Services by the National Development Group for the Mentally Han-

dicapped, Department of Health and Social Security, 1978.
Toy Library Association, Seabrook House, Wyllyotts Manor,
Darkes Lane, Potters Bar, Herts.

Downs Childrens Association, Old Rectory, Honeywood Walk,
Carshalton, Surrey *or*:
Downs Childrens Association, Quinborne Community Centre,
Ridgacre Road, Quinton, Birmingham 32.

Derbyshire Language Scheme.
> Details of Training Courses from Mr M. Masidlover,
> Educational Psychologist, Area Education Office,
> Grosvenor Road, Ripley, Derby.

Reference for Developmental Progress

Children's Developmental Progress: from birth to five years: the Stycar Sequences by Mary D. Sheridan (Published by NFER Windsor.)
> One of the most comprehensive and detailed scales of
> developmental progress, covering: visual competence, hear-
> ing and listening, communication and motor development.
> Although the progress is given in normal milestones, these
> can easily be related to mental ages. This book is a 'must' for
> anyone working with children of all ages.

Books on Feeding

Handling the Young Cerebral Palsied Child at Home, by Nancy Finnie. (Published by Heinemann.)
> Very good section on feeding.

Feeding Can be Fun, by Mary Ryan. (Published by Spastics Society (Publications Department), 12 Park Crescent, London W1N 4 EQ.)
> Very inexpensive and practical booklet.

'Feeding Techniques with Cerebral Palsied Children', by J. Blockley and G. Millar. (Published in *Physiotherapy Journal*, April, May, June 1971, pp. 300–8.)

Books and Information on Autism

Early Childhood Autism (2nd Edn). Edited by Dr L. Wing. (Published by Pergamon Press, 1976.)

'Language communication and the use of symbols in normal and autistic children', by Derek M. Ricks and L. Wing. (Published in *Journal of Autism and Childhood Schizophrenia, Vol.* 5, 3, 1975.)

An Approach to Teaching Autistic Children. Edited by M. P. Everard. (Published by Pergamon Press.)

Conferences, Seminars, Training Courses, etc.

British Institute of Mental Handicap, Wolverhampton Road, Kidderminster, Worcs.
> Membership of Institute recommended. Wide variety of conferences and seminars available on subjects of interest in mental handicap.

National Hospitals College of Speech Sciences (Hampstead Branch), 84a Heath Street, Hampstead, London NW3 1DN.
> Wide variety of courses held on subjects related to communication.

Castle Priory College, Thames Street, Wallingford, Oxfordshire OX10 0HE.
> Full programme of courses on wide variety of subjects including mental handicap.

National Society for Mentally Handicapped Children, 117 Golden Lane, London EC1 0RT.
> Variety of courses held on subjects related to mental handicap.

Speech Therapy Services

If your establishment does not have a speech therapist and advice is required, contact your area speech therapist through the Area Health Authority Offices. Or contact the speech therapist at your district hospital or local health centre, and she will inform you of the recommended procedure.

Alternative Means of Communication

The Makaton Vocabulary

For information and details of training courses, contact: Mrs M. Walker, Project Co-Ordinator, Makaton Vocabulary Development Project, 85 Pierrefondes Avenue, Farnborough, Hants.

Paget-Gorman Sign System

For information and details of training courses, contact: Field Officer, Paget-Gorman Sign System, Centre for the Deaf, The City Lit., Keeley House, Keeley Street, London WC2B 4BA.

Blissymbolics Communication

For information and details of training courses, contact: Mrs E. Davies, National Adviser, Blissymbolics Communication Research Centre (UK), South Glamorgan Institute of Higher Education, Western Avenue, Llandaff, Cardiff CF5 2YB.

11

EDUCATION OF THE SEVERELY MENTALLY HANDICAPPED

N. B. Crawford

DEVELOPMENT OF EDUCATIONAL SERVICES PRIOR TO 1971

Moderate Subnormality

The Education Act (1944) introduced the term 'educationally sub-normal' to describe children 'who by reason of limited ability or other conditions resulting in educational retardation, require some specialised form of education wholly or partly in substitution for the education normally given in ordinary schools', and these were estimated at 5–10% of the school population. Special schools were designated for this purpose and referred to as ESN schools. Although 'intelligence quotients' as such are not mentioned, the quotients of children placed at ESN schools were generally between 50 and 70.

Severe Mental Subnormality

In the early part of this century, severe mental handicap was seen as a permanent and unchanging state: 'Amentia is a permanent condition which calls for permanent care' (1923 Annual Report of Board of Control). Little significant progress appears to have been

175

achieved until the 1950s and 1960s when the work of people like Tizard, O'Connor, Hermelin and Gunzberg began to have an impact.

Further impetus to change came with the 1959 Mental Health Act. Part 2, section 11 replaced section 57 of the Education Act 1944 and made it a duty for local education authorities to ascertain those children who were unsuitable for education in school by virtue of 'disability of mind', and were empowered to compel the medical examination of any child from the age of 2 years. In section 12 the local health authority was empowered to compel regular attendance of severely mentally handicapped children of school age at junior training centres, but because of the shortage of such centres in most parts of the country these powers of compulsion were rarely invoked.

In 1970 the Education (Handicapped Children) Act was introduced which transferred responsibility from Local Health to the Education Department making it the duty of the latter to provide education for all children, including the severely subnormal. The severely mentally handicapped were, therefore, in 1971 the last group of children to be brought within the education system.

As a result of this legislation, the Department of Education and Science (DES) assumed responsibility for the education of about 20 000 children in junior training centres and about 8000 children in hospital schools. These were referred to as ESN(S) schools to distinguish them from those for the moderately subnormal ESN(M) schools which were already in existence. The incidence of severe subnormality up to 16 years was estimated to be not less than four per thousand (DES, 1975).

The Warnock Report (1978) states:

> Organisational changes and additional resources will not be sufficient in themselves to achieve our aims. They must be accompanied by changes in attitude. Special education must be seen as a form of educational activity no less important, no less demanding and no less rewarding than any other, and teachers, administrators and other professionals engaged in it must have the same commitment to children with special needs as they have to other children.

IMPLICATIONS OF THE TRANSFER FROM HEALTH TO EDUCATION

Staff Training

One of the major implications for the DES was staff training. Less than half the teachers in junior training centres, and less than a quarter of the teachers in the existing hospital schools were qualified (Bland, 1968) and the Scott Report (1962) argued strongly for training courses of at least two years. Unqualified staff in the newly adopted special schools were offered the opportunity to achieve qualified status by taking the Diploma in the Education of Mentally Handicapped Children (Dip. NAMH), followed by a period of probation. The last course for this qualification was held in 1972/3. Since that time, teachers in ESN(S) schools take the standard teacher training courses which in some colleges lay emphasis on the education of mentally handicapped children.

Methods of Teaching and Curricula

Allied to staff training, it was recognized that there was a need to develop methods of teaching and establish standardized curricula. Initially the essentially occupational activities in use were replaced by certain nursery/infant methods which later proved to be unsuitable, through the experience of practice and in various research studies.

Buildings

Many junior training centre buildings which were not purpose-built have had to be modified to meet changing needs, and since 1971 many new purpose-built centres have been provided to replace older inadequate facilities. In addition, hospital school buildings have been modernized or replaced by new buildings and this has been accompanied by efforts to place as many severely mentally handicapped children as possible in schools outside.

PRESENT PROVISIONS

We shall be concerned here with the group described as severely subnormal. Section 4(2) of the Mental Health Act (1959) described severe subnormality as:

> a state of arrested or incomplete development of mind, which includes subnormality of intelligence, and is of such a nature or degree that the patient is incapable of living an independent life or guarding himself against serious exploitation, or will be so incapable when of an age to do so.

The majority of ESN(S) schools cater for the full age range from 5 to 16 years which is the statutory school-leaving age, although some local education authorities are providing places for children below 5 and above 18 years of age.

IDENTIFICATION AND NOTIFICATION OF MENTAL HANDICAP

Identification of handicap usually takes place at the paediatric assessment and developmental units in general hospitals at which most children are born. Children may also be referred to these units by health visitors and general practitioners.

In most parts of the United Kingdom a system of notification to social service and education departments has been established when the diagnosis has been confirmed, so that as soon as a child is identified these departments are aware of the need and can then provide very early support and guidance services.

MENTAL HANDICAP HOSPITALS

Some 50 000 people are at present in mental handicap hospitals in the United Kingdom; of these people, about 3000 are under 16 years of age. Most hospitals for the mentally handicapped now have well-staffed schools attached, with access to multidisciplinary expertise, and are in a position to serve three particular needs:

1. multidisciplinary assessment, either through daily attendance or while the child is resident;
2. regular review of medication and other forms of treatment;
3. education for the most severely mentally and multiply handicapped children who require medical and nursing care and

those who show grossly hyperactive or bizarre behaviour patterns.

Primary and Secondary ESN(S) Schools

Some local authorities have separated the older ESN(S) children from the younger ones by arranging for the older children from about the age of 12 to attend a secondary ESN(S) school; these schools often provide full-time education up to the age of 18 years.

Integration

Occasionally ESN(M) and (S) children have been integrated into one school, although this is rare. Never have large numbers of severely handicapped children been integrated into ordinary schools.

Involvement of Specialists

Increasingly, especially in schools outside hospitals, educational psychologists, as a part of the psychological services to schools, are becoming involved in the methods of teaching and training employed rather than being used purely for psychological testing. Schools in hospitals usually have the help of clinical psychologists, both for testing and in the application of behaviour modification. Speech therapists, who have traditionally carried out individual treatment programmes, are now also advising on the design and implementation of language programmes and methods of communication within the schools.

Additional visiting specialists may also include psychiatrists, physiotherapists, teachers for the hearing-impaired and for the visually handicapped. Some local authorities have the advantage of a number of community nurses specializing in schoolchildren and their families, in conjunction with social workers who provide a mechanism for increasing the effectiveness of home–school relations.

An interesting account of the provisions of one local authority is given by Rhys-Jones (1973).

179

CURRICULUM DEVELOPMENT

There are currently a variety of approaches to the curricula operating within the ESN(S) schools, and from a review of the literature the reader will gather that at the present time an eclectic approach is commonplace.

Research

In the Brooklands (1964) experiment a group of children using nursery-school facilities were found to improve greatly on verbal measures compared with a control group in hospital. However, there was no difference on non-verbal measures and this often-overlooked aspect of the experiment may have contributed to the initial use of nursery and infant methods to the teaching of severely subnormal children. This is, however, now generally regarded as contrary to evidence from research on the learning processes of the handicapped as, although normal infants appear to learn spontaneously in a stimulating environment, the handicapped child does not necessarily learn from his environment but requires it to be far more structured. Clarke and Clarke (1974) offer a useful survey of research in this area. It follows that an enriched environment is not enough on its own, and both the surroundings and the stimulation provided must be organized and structured to be of benefit to the severely subnormal. It must also be remembered that, although superficially the mental ages of handicapped children may suggest that methods and materials transferred from infant school curricula are appropriate, the emotional and social needs of severely subnormal children are likely to be nearer their chronological than their mental age.

Guidelines for Present Practices

There are at least two important lessons for teachers, and these lessons are supported through experience and research. First, a high degree of structure is required in teaching, coupled with clear objectives and small incremental steps to enable handicapped students to learn more effectively. It is also clear that the removal of irrelevant stimuli is very relevant. An association between these essentials for effective learning and common areas of difficulty in the mentally handicapped, e.g. input, storage or recall, are, as yet, unclear.

Secondly, the application of behavioural techniques in training programmes has been effectively demonstrated, both in the USA and the UK. The behavioural approach concentrates on clearly stated unambiguous objectives, the arrangement of reinforcement, the conditions under which the behaviour is to occur and the criteria by means of which it can be agreed that a specific objective has been achieved (Gronlund, 1970). This approach encourages careful structuring and the use of one to one teaching.

A DES pamphlet (1975) states that 'many successful practices are based on theories of operant conditioning', and emphasizes the importance of clear statements of objectives and indicates current good practices using this approach.

A fuller discussion of these principles will be found in the chapter on the behavioural approach. Developmental charts of achievement are in common use in schools in a variety of forms, e.g. Progress Assessment Charts (PAC), Sheridan, Portage, etc. However, there are a number of problems related to many developmental checklists which have not been specially designed for classroom use. They are concerned with skills displayed in normal children, their observed order of appearance primarily providing a method by means of which individual children may be compared.

The steps in many checklists do not readily lend themselves to teaching for a number of reasons: many are too large; not all are essential; and there are a number of steps missing in data obtained from normal children which are essential for handicapped children. The latter may also have abnormalities and are, therefore, not likely to follow the normal pattern and sequence of development.

SCHOOL-BASED CURRICULA

Many schools, rather than using a prepared curriculum, are producing their own, and involve teachers both in design and implementation. All ESN(S) schools should include the following as priorities:

1. *Self-help.* Toileting; feeding; undressing; dressing; washing. (See Appendix I.)
2. *Communication.* The development of language, of a receptive and an expressive vocabulary; the possible use of a signing system (e.g. Paget-Gorman or Makaton) or a symbol system (e.g. Rebus or Bliss); the ability to read social sight words such as toilet, poison, push, etc.
3. *Motor development.* Motor development, such as walking, running, jumping; the development of movements leading to a greater awareness of self, of body image; the training of fine motor skills and co-ordination.
4. *Social education.* A broad heading which may be subdivided to include:
   (a) shopping;
   (b) domestic work;
   (c) leisure;
   (d) mobility (including using transport in the community);
   (e) cooking;
   (f) self-care and hygiene;
   (g) interpersonal and sexual relationships.
5. *Training in safety.* The training to develop safe habits in everyday life:
   (a) at home: using electrical appliances, care with common poisonous substances, gas, fire, etc;
   (b) at work: what to do in the event of an accident, dangers of sharp objects, protective and sensible clothing;
   (c) in the community: dangers of traffic and training in road safety, who to ask for help, who not to accept lifts or help from, etc.
6. *Vocational training.* Developing good work habits, time-keeping, specified work skills.

In addition to these 'core areas' (Crawford, 1980) such subjects as art, craft, music, swimming, horse-riding, educational visits and other extramural activities should also be considered to widen experience. It is up to the individual school to decide its own priorities, and each pupil should follow a specific programme designed to meet his/her own special needs. It should also be the function of the school to meet these needs and to enable the parents not just to be aware of the progress of their child but to be actively involved in it at every opportunity.

SPECIAL CARE

Reference has already been made to the fact that there are more children in this category in hospital schools than in day schools for the ESN(S). In many schools, however, there are now classes or departments designed to provide for the most severely handicapped. Such children are generally grossly physically handicapped and non-ambulant, and frequently require help with feeding, dressing and toileting.

Teaching programmes designed for these children must take into account their additional handicaps. It will also be necessary for special furniture and equipment to be available or constructed to assist in their management. Special chairs, tables, feeding aids, specially designed spoon handles, plate guards and non-slip mats, for example, might be used. It is essential that there are short periods of intensive individual training, and that limitations on their teaching are not too readily placed on them because of their apparent intellectual level. In many ESN(S) schools since 1971 it has been found that an initial low expectation can become a self-fulfilling prophecy. The environment and life of these children needs to be structured but stimulating and changing. If, for instance, the child is not ambulant he must be moved to new areas of interest, and even if cot-bound for part of the day the use of different mobiles or pictures on the ceiling is important. In this area the advice of specialist staff, such as occupational therapists and physiotherapists, can be invaluable. Assessments and a knowledge of the baseline abilities of each child with an indication of his/her physical disabilities are essential.

Occasionally, the term 'special care' is also used to refer to those children who are extremely disruptive and many of whom also show other forms of bizarre behaviour, including psychotic features. Such children need to be managed and treated in small groups with additional staff, and advice will be required from psychiatrists and psychologists.

It should be pointed out that, although it is said that there are some advantages in placing children with similar problems together, these advantages usually relate to the similarity of the programmes used with them and the ease of organization. If modelling, however, is to be regarded as an effective teaching technique, then it follows that for children to be exposed to mixed-ability groups enables them to model more acceptable behaviours in those around them. It should always be the ultimate aim to integrate the children, even for short periods, with their less handicapped peers.

FURTHER EDUCATION

It has long been felt that the handicapped require an extended period of education, as the majority are likely to be 'slow learners'. All now remain at school until they are 16 years of age, and some until they are 18 years of age, before leaving to attend adult training centres. Schools should prepare them for placement in adult training centres by sampling the work done, regular visits by part-time phasing-in during the last few weeks of school life. Education should continue at the adult training centre where the emphasis should be on social training – in fact, training and experience for work if possible and life in general.

It is vital that properly designed programmes are implemented in adult training centres to enable them to meet the objectives decided. There is now a good deal of evidence which supports continued training (Baranyay, 1971).

The extent to which adult education for the mentally handicapped is available varies from one area to another. Some courses may be offered at a further education college, community schools and centres, and at technical colleges in addition to the adult training centres; for further details see the chapter on training in adult units.

THE FUTURE

It has always taken a number of years for evidence from research to be applied in the classroom. At present some educationists only see the behavioural approach as a technique for modifying undesirable behaviour and do not recognize its wider implications for the learning of skills which can be broken down and taught in

184

simple small steps (Crawford, Gardner and Murphy, 1980).

Schools should become more concerned with the production of a clear and positive statement of their objectives on each child and the means by which they may be achieved.

School-based curricula will require in-service staff training to bring about changes in attitude and a greater awareness of the techniques of evaluation. Any assumptions regarding the efficacy of methods should be thoroughly examined, and evaluation must go hand in hand with curriculum changes. Ongoing staff discussion on curricula and their evaluation will not only ensure greater involvement but also provide for the development of professional expertise.

Movement of Children out of Mental Handicap Hospitals

Although there are still 3000 children in hospitals, few are being admitted for permanent care and many of those who are there cannot be discharged because appropriate care is not available elsewhere; it is to be hoped, however, that such children will ultimately find their way into community homes. Hospitals of the future are likely to cater only for those who need continuous medical (including psychiatric) and nursing care, and for some who require long-term assessment. This change in approach in recent years is a very significant and important one, and will also require a considerable change in attitude and approach of the staff of all ESN(S) schools in the community.

Bibliography

Baranyay, E. (1971). *The Mentally Handicapped Adolescent*. (Oxford: Pergamon Press)

Bland, G. A. (1968). *Education in Hospital Schools for the Mentally Handicapped*. (London: National Council for Special Education)

Clarke, A. D. B. and Clarke, A. M. (1974). *The Changing Outlook*. (London: Methuen)

Crawford, N. B (1980). *Curriculum Planning*, No. 1. (Kidderminster: British Institute of Mental Handicap)

Crawford, N. B., Gardner, J. M. and Murphy, J. (1980). *The Skills Analysis Model: an Effective Curriculum for Severely Educationally Subnormal Children*. (Kidderminster: British Institute of Mental Handicap) (In press)

DES (1975). *Educating Mentally Handicapped Children.* Pamphlet No. 60. (London: HMSO)

Griffiths, M. (1973). *The Young Retarded Child.* (Edinburgh: Churchill Livingstone)

Gronlund, N. (1970). *Stating Behavioural Objectives for Classroom Instruction.* (London: Macmillan)

Rhys-Jones, W. G. (1973). Community Services, In *The Young Retarded Child,* chap. 6, pp. 62–70 (London: Macmillan)

Scott Report (1962). The Training of Staff of Training Centres for the Mentally Handicapped. (London: HMSO)

Tizard, J. (1964). *Community Services for the Mentally Handicapped,* pp. 85–130. (London: Oxford University Press)

Warnock Report (1978). Report of the Committee of Enquiry into Education of the Handicapped Children and Young People. (London: HMSO)

Further Reading

Bender, M. and Valletutti, P. (1977). *Teaching the Moderately and Severely Handicapped.* (Baltimore: University Park Press)

DHSS (1970). *Transfer of Responsibility for the Education of Mentally Handicapped Children.* (London: HMSO)

DHSS (1971). *Better Services for the Mentally Handicapped.* (London: HMSO)

Guidelines for Teachers No. 9. (1971). *Backward over 100 years.* (London: National Council for Special Education)

Mittler, P. (1970). *The Psychological Assessment of Mental and Physical Handicaps.* (London: Methuen)

Pritchard, D. G. (1963). *Education and the Handicapped (1760–1960).* (London: Routledge & Kegan Paul)

APPENDIX I

Name of Student: ....
CURRICULUM AREA: SELF CARE

K. Target Behaviour: Clean shoes correctly
Criterion: St. will carry out procedures on three consecutive trials without any prompt.
Conditions: Using polish, brushes (pads, cream), cloths, collecting own items.
Rewards used:

Start date								
1. Point to utensils when named								
2. Collect utensils (listed)								
3. Remove mud from shoes, either onto newspaper or outside								
4. Dispose of newspaper								
5. Lay fresh newspaper on table or floor								
6. Smear polish on shoe with cloth								
7. Polish off with shoebrush								
8. Final shine with pad								
9. Put shoes away								
10. Dispose of newspaper								
11. Wash and dry hands								

Code used: V: verbal prompt; G: gestural prompt; P: physical prompt; ✓: behaviour performed correctly without prompts.

Note: This is a worksheet forming part of a social education programme. It illustrates the need for structure in the teaching and recording of work with ESN(S) pupils. Each of the behaviours listed may require separate programmes or the step-size between skills may be reduced for certain children. This extract is from the Social Education Programme in use at the Mary Elliot School in Walsall, West Midlands.

12

TRAINING, EMPLOYMENT AND RECREATIONAL ACTIVITIES FOR ADULTS

M. Phillips

ADULT TRAINING CENTRES

In the United Kingdom the provision of day services for mentally handicapped adults is the responsibility of the Social Services Department of the area in which the person resides, and this has been provided mainly in the form of adult training centres (ATCs). In addition, there are a number of other facilities for adults which may be provided by local education authorities, through their further education departments, and by voluntary bodies.

Although the development of these services has received a high priority both from central and local government during the past 20 years, there are still waiting lists in many parts of the country and the shortage of places for school-leavers has increased in the past 3 years.

MANAGEMENT AND STAFFING OF ADULT TRAINING CENTRES

Each centre has a manager supported by instructors, some of whom have the Diploma in Training and Education of Mentally

189

Handicapped Adults and some of whom may be qualified teachers. From 1981 the appropriate qualification for staff in ATCs will be the Certificate in Social Services awarded by the Central Council for Education and Training in Social Work (CCETSW).

The manager is usually accountable to an assistant director with responsibility for day services in the Social Services Department and should be in regular contact with a principal officer from this division.

In authorities which have decentralized the management of their services to areas or divisions, closer links have been established between the ATC staff and the local field and residential staff, which should result in families getting a more co-ordinated service.

SHIFT IN THE EMPHASIS OF PROGRAMMES AT ATCs

There has been a considerable shift of emphasis at ATCs in the last decade from industrial and contract work (largely assembly, dismantling and packaging) to the development of a more broadly based programme which includes social training, basic education with some industrial or horticultural work when it is appropriate to the individual. The National Development Group Pamphlet No. 5, *Day Services for Mentally Handicapped Adults,* provides useful guidelines for the development of good practice in ATCs.

THE ALLOCATION OF PLACES AND SCHOOL-LEAVERS' CONFERENCES

The allocation of places at ATCs usually takes place through discussion at school-leavers' conferences which are held during the last or penultimate year spent at the special school. These conferences are usually organized by the Education Authorities and attended by representatives of the Social Services Department and Health Authority. In some areas, parents are also invited so that they may become involved to a greater extent in the plans being made for their children's future.

TRANSITION PROGRAMMES

In many areas transition programmes are arranged which enable pupils to spend a day each week, possibly increasing to 2-3 days each week, at the ATC during their last year at school. In addition to providing those about to be moved with an opportunity to become accustomed to the new environment, it also helps the staff of the special school, and the centre, to learn more about each other's work; this results in a more co-ordinated service.

SCHOOL LEAVING AGE

Until 1975 it was the practice for most mentally handicapped pupils to leave special schools at 16 years of age. Since then there has been increasing recognition of the fact that many mentally handicapped 16-year-olds (whose mental age will be considerably lower) do benefit from remaining at school until 18 or 19 years of age, and because of the drop in the birth rate in some parts of the country, education authorities have been able to keep them longer at school. In addition, in some areas 'senior special schools' have been set up which are providing a very appropriate syllabus for mentally handicapped pupils of 13-18 years of age.

TRAINING FOR STAFF

The slower learning rate of the mentally handicapped, and their special needs in learning and the paucity of experience, makes it important for the teachers involved in the special schools and the training staff of centres to co-ordinate their programmes and exchange information whatever the age at which transfer takes place. Some authorities have found it very helpful to organize joint in-service training courses for teachers and ATC staff and to invite ATC staff to attend courses organized for staff of special schools and colleges of further education.

CONTENT OF TRAINING

Assessment, Programming and Review

All training programmes should start with a comprehensive assessment, linked to regular reviews involving all the staff concerned

191

with the programme, and the family (see chapters on Behaviour, Communication and Sensory and Motor Handicap for information on the details of assessment). More attention is now being paid in ATCs to assessment, review and the recording of progress. To a great extent the realization of the individual's potential and the development of stimulating programmes is dependent on staff acquiring skills in these areas.

Social Training

The increasing recognition of the importance of providing experience and training aimed at independent living has led to the development of social training schemes in many ATCs. Unfortunately, many ATCs were built at a time when a more limited view of the potential of mentally handicapped people was taken and did not include the appropriate facilities for social training in this area. However, many of these buildings have been adapted with ingenuity and imagination to provide flats and accommodation for teaching in small groups.

Work Preparation

The current emphasis on the importance of a broadly based programme focusing on social training should not be at the expense of preparation and training for employment for those able to benefit and with the potential to obtain employment. This experience may be provided either in an advanced work section or in a separate building designed for industrial training where normal working conditions can be simulated. In addition to intensive training in specific skills, programmes should also include the ability to travel on public transport and attendance for normal working hours. In addition, there should be an educational element to enable trainees to learn about employers' expectations, national insurance, income tax matters and trade union membership.

Motivation and Reward

Motivation to train and work is as important to the mentally handicapped as to any other member of society. The individual needs to experience satisfaction from what he is doing and also receive monetary reward which he or she can regard as an appropriate recompense for achievement. It is obviously not always realistic for rewards to be associated only with output, as the latter may be so limited in the case of the severely handicapped as to be negligible despite the fact that it is all the individual is able to achieve.

It is essential for staff to ensure that trainees are adequately rewarded on their output. Factors such as effort, punctuality and behaviour should also be taken into account. These aspects must be assessed, not against the performance of non-handicapped persons but in terms of the handicapped person's own capabilities and potential. This makes the initial assessment and subsequent reviews of great importance in helping trainees to reach attainable goals.

HEALTH SERVICES

Although day-care services for adults are the responsibility of Social Services Departments, there is a need for a number of medical and para-medical services similar to those provided at special schools which at present tend to cease on leaving school. These services are essential for the mentally handicapped who are entitled to all the facilities available to the general public.

Whilst physiotherapists, speech therapists and chiropodists may be in too short supply to provide sessions for individuals, they should be able at least to give ATC staff advice, guidance and support in these areas. In addition, regular sessions from psychiatrists and clinical psychologists to help develop methods of assessment and curriculum planning, with advice on the use of the behavioural approach to training and the management of behaviour problems, should be available.

To an increasing extent, as consultants in mental handicap and members of specialist mental handicap teams are providing support services to families, they should be regarded as members of the extended team of the ATC so that it is not left to the initiative of parents alone to try to obtain these essential services.

Dental officers and health visitors should be available for dental care and personal hygiene, whilst the advice of a dietician may also be useful.

TRANSPORT AND MEALS

Most authorities provide free transport to the centre from home or a nearby pick-up point although, in some areas, trainees have to spend up to an hour and a half each day on the coach. The staff of some centres undertake a 'travel training' programme with the help of parents, which enables the more able to use public transport not only to reach the centre but also for their leisure and social activities. A mid-day meal is also provided at the centre, for which a charge is made. The arrangements for the meal can provide opportunities for social training and the development of self-help skills.

SPECIAL CARE UNITS

Until comparatively recently there has been some uncertainty as to whether the multiply handicapped and the most severely dependent people should be catered for in ATCs. A greater realization of the capacity of these individuals to respond to training and stimulation, as a result of the work done in units for them at special schools and in some hospitals, has resulted in a considerable change of attitude. All that has already been said about the provision of health services is of even greater importance for the special care units.

It is now generally accepted that each ATC should provide for the most severely handicapped and that staff will need to be very skilled and well supported. (The National Development Group have recommended minimum staffing ratio of 1 : 3.) Both the handicapped and the staff benefit from being part of an adult training unit, and there should always be the possibility of movement for staff and trainees between the special care unit and other sections of the centre.

DEPARTMENT OF EMPLOYMENT

The Department's employment and training services are now run by the Employment Service Agency and the Training Service Agency under the Manpower Services Commission.

Disablement Resettlement Officers (DROs) are based at local employment offices and job centres to advise and help handicapped people on local employment possibilities and training facilities available throughout the community. They also encourage employers to take on disabled people, giving advice and support. Assessment courses provide guidance as to an individual's suitability for various types of work or training. Employment rehabilitation courses designed to help handicapped people to adjust to normal working conditions are available.

Disabled Persons Register

Handicapped people over the age of 18 years who are capable of employment may seek registration on the disabled persons register at the local employment office or job centre. The main advantages are opportunities of participating in suitable training schemes. Some sheltered employment is only open to people on the register, and certain employers have a statutory obligation to employ a quota of registered disabled persons (although this is frequently not enforced).

Sheltered Employment

Local authorities are empowered, under the Disabled Persons (Employment) Act 1958, to set up workshops for severely disabled people. Central government provides financial help in the form of grants towards trading losses, capital expenditure and training. Relatively few authorities have set up sheltered workshops and those that have, have usually to provide for the full range of handicapped people; the number of severely mentally handicapped people taken on is small. Some authorities have developed multipurpose centres (i.e. sheltered workshops, adult training centres and day centres for physically handicapped), partly to make it easier for people to transfer from one section to another.

Enclaves

This is a group of severely disabled people working together under special supervision in an ordinary working environment. The Employment Services Agency approves the scheme in ad /ance and is involved in the selection of employees. The enclaves must be run by a non-profit-making organization, i.e. a local authority or voluntary organization.

Payments of up to 75% between the difference in earned and paid wages may be made by the Employment Services Agency in addition to allowances for administrative costs, including the supervisor's salary. Such schemes involve the local authority in at least 25% of the cost of the project.

Those authorities who have set up enclaves have used them for providing a meals-on-wheels kitchen, or a laundry service for residential or day-care services, or employment in parks and gardens.

Liaison with Trade Unions

A committee, which includes representatives of a community health council, educationalists and trade unionists, started a campaign in 1977 in a large city to increase and encourage employment opportunities for mentally handicapped people (East Birmingham CHC, 203 Bordesley Green East, Birmingham). As a result of this, many of the difficulties frequently experienced over the level of wages and attitudes of other workers may be overcome.

FINANCE

At the age of 16 years, or at the upper limit of compulsory school age, every mentally handicapped person not in employment is entitled to a weekly income through supplementary benefit. He/she is also entitled to apply for a range of discretionary benefits to cover bedding, clothing and heating. Exceptional needs, due to poor health and restricted mobility, may qualify for additional allowances. Application should be made to the local Department of Health and Social Security office (Forms SB1 are also available in Post Offices). Children over 16 years of age in full-time education who are so handicapped as to make employment at school-leaving age unlikely, are also able to claim supplementary benefit.

In deciding the amounts of benefit the income of the parents is not taken into account. Mobility and attendance allowances are disregarded but NCIP is taken fully into account. The first £4 of any weekly earnings, after deducting fares and associated expenses, is also disregarded. Further information can be obtained from the *'Disability Rights Handbook for 1979'*, The Disability Alliance, 5 Netherhall Gardens, London NW3 5RJ.

FURTHER EDUCATION

The fact that a young person attends an ATC should not mean that he or she is not eligible for further education on a part-time or day-release basis. To an increasing extent, further education colleges are providing links and other special courses for people attending ATCs. In some instances they may attend courses already running for non-handicapped people, and participate in adult literacy programmes which are available at many colleges and centres of adult education.

Further education can be provided in a variety of ways. It is important that the arrangements and the content of programmes are known and agreed by the staff of the ATC who are responsible for the major part of the individual's learning programme.

LEISURE AND RECREATION

The emphasis on the handicap, rather than the recognition of their potential and the tendency of parents and staff to adopt an over-protective attitude towards mentally handicapped adults, may result in their leading very circumscribed social lives. In fact, they have the same ability to enjoy themselves as the rest of the community. Many are very sociable and show an interest in sport, music, art and crafts.

Whilst there are a range of leisure activities specially designed for the mentally handicapped it is important that full advantage should be taken of facilities available to the general public, in order that they can become fully integrated into the community. The mentally handicapped may need help in making use of facilities such as leisure centres, swimming baths, public libraries and community centres, just as other members of society may need assistance in accepting them as individuals in their own right.

SERVICES PROVIDED BY VOLUNTARY ORGANIZATIONS

National Society for Mentally Handicapped Children (NSMHC)

The National Society for Mentally Handicapped Children runs residential courses at three centres for school-leavers and young moderately and severely handicapped adults. The cost of these courses is usually borne by the sponsoring authority. Apart from the vocational content of the course, the centres focus on developing each individual's potential for independence, in relation to employment, daily living and social behaviour. At the end of the course it is the responsibility of the sponsoring authority, in conjunction with the local employment service, to help place the young person in suitable employment. It is important for staff from the home area to keep in close touch with the staff at the centre and with the mentally handicapped person and his family throughout the period of the course.

The three centres are:

1. *Dilston Hall, Northumberland:* an advanced social training unit. This unit provides a programme of work experience and an opportunity to learn how to get along with other people and develop social experience (the course duration is usually 2 years).
2. *Lufton Manor Rural Training Unit, Yeovil:* provides 2-year full-time training in horticulture and agriculture.
3. *Pengwern Hall, Rhuddlan:* an experimental unit which provides transition training to equip young people to cope with the demands of normal living and work situations. The emphasis is on self-help in daily living.

Pathway Scheme, South Wales

This scheme provides training for mentally handicapped people in sponsored employment using 'foster workers' for a period of 6 months. The trainees' wages and the fee/honorarium paid to the foster workers are paid by the local NSMHC who also employ a Regional Placement Officer whose responsibility includes:

1. assessment of trainee's readiness for employment;
2. finding and preparing employers and foster workers;
3. supporting the trainee and staff during the placement.

Whilst there is no commitment on the employer to retain the trainee at the end of the period, the majority have done so. The scheme originated in South Wales and because of its success in placing mentally handicapped people in employment, the NSMHC have decided to encourage other regions to appoint Placement Officers to develop similar schemes.

Training in Horticulture

Because of the interest shown by local authorities in the horticultural training at Lufton Manor, the NSMHC have set up an Advisory Service for Rural Training (Director: Mr D. Carter, 100 High Street, Yatton, Bristol). As a result a number of local authorities have been able to extend their ATC programmes to include a systematic training in horticulture and marketing of produce. This applies equally to urban areas where there is possibility of employment in the Parks and Gardens Department.

Training in Agriculture

Other local authorities are developing farm training schemes based on the experience gained at Lufton (e.g. Buckinghamshire has received a grant from the Harding Education Charity to finance a special course for eight or nine mentally handicapped students at a local authority college farm. Hampshire is also developing a project with the help of NSMHC Advisory Service.)

National Federation of Gateway Clubs

The NSMHC has appointed a National Officer to help with the development of local Gateway clubs. The Federation also runs courses for club leaders. Club meetings are usually held weekly and weekend activities, including sport and outings, are also organized. In some places the club is held at the local ATC and provides a close link between parents, staff and volunteers. In other places the local NSMHC has provided its own centre.

Holidays

The NSMHC also runs a variety of holiday facilities which offer accommodation for individuals with or without their families and for groups.

Many local societies have bought their own caravans or chalets which are let to families, giving priority to their own members. *Parents Voice* (the quarterly magazine published by the NSMHC) often includes advertisements for holidays of this kind.

Staff at many ATCs organize and raise funds each year to enable them to take trainees on very enterprising holidays. These range from holiday camps in the country and youth hostelling to trips abroad and outward bound schemes. For instance, a centre in Wales enables trainees to participate in mountain-climbing and pony-trekking. Centres also participate in football, swimming and athletics competitions which are now usually run on a regional and inter-regional basis.

COMMUNITY SERVICE

Mentally handicapped people enjoy being of service to others and our desire to provide a good-quality service for them should not deprive them of the opportunity of helping others should they wish to do so. Obviously, very careful preparation and selection of appropriate services and the individuals involved is important, but the results invariably justify the amount of work involved, both for the mentally handicapped themselves and those who are being helped.

A good example of a scheme to prepare mentally handicapped people for community service as part of an ATC programme can be found at the Old Sarum Adult Training Centre, Salisbury, where 80% of the trainees spend half a day on some form of community service, but there are many other ATCs now carrying out similar programmes.

CONFERENCES FOR THE MENTALLY HANDICAPPED

Campaign for the Mentally Handicapped has run a series of participatory events, including one-day events and several residential conferences for mentally handicapped adults living at home or in hostels or hospital. Participants are encouraged to discuss their experiences of the services they receive and the services they would like. In this way they develop more confidence in their ability to communicate with other people. The programmes also include a range of activities such as music-making, painting and craft work, drama and dancing, which are shared by the non-handicapped. Further information can be obtained from Campaign for the Mentally Handicapped, Publications, 8 Church End, Gamlingay, Sandy, Bedfordshire.

WORKERS EDUCATIONAL ASSOCIATION (WEA)

The WEA is an independent voluntary movement run by its members and recognized by the Department of Education and Science for the provision of adult education. The Department makes it a grant which enables each of the 21 districts to employ full- and part-time staff. The WEA has a traditional concern for the under-privileged and in recent years has become increasingly involved in educational work for socially deprived and handicapped people, including those who are in long-stay hospitals or homes, i.e. those who might not otherwise be offered adult education. One of the aims in providing education to handicapped people is to help them develop their self-respect. A comprehensive programme is now organized in the Western Region for mentally handicapped adults living in hospitals, hostels or at home.

Reading List

Day Services for Mentally Handicapped Adults. National Development Group Pamphlet No. 5 (London: DHSS)

Employment Services Agency (1976). *Employing Someone who is Mentally Handicapped*

Employment Services Agency (1976). *Rehabilitation, Resettlement and Employment Services for Handicapped People*

King Edward's Hospital Fund (1973). *A Library Service for the Mentally Handicapped.* (M.H. Papers 3)

King Edward's Hospital Fund (1975). *Adult Education for Mentally Handicapped People* (M.H. Papers 3) Mental Handicap Paper 3

Whelan, E. and Speake, B., *Adult Training Centres in England and Wales*: (Manchester: University of Manchester Press)

NSMHC literature relating to Gateway Clubs and holiday facilities

Campaign for Mentally Handicapped publications on employment and participation

Sheffield Evaluation Reseach Group: *Study on Adult Training Centres*

13

PARENTS' NEEDS AND HOW TO MEET THEM

Leslie Marks

'It is only very recently that the needs of mentally handicapped children and their families have begun to receive the
attention they deserve. The time is not long gone when, once
the diagnosis was established, parents were left very much to
their own devices. . .' (Day, 1977)

COPING WITH HANDICAP

Immediate Effects of Birth

The birth of a mentally handicapped child is a devastating experience. It follows a period of preparation and joyful anticipation
– which is suddenly brought to a full stop. Usually it is an event
totally outside the experience of everyone concerned. It threatens
the whole being of the parents, and shatters the hopes vested in the
unborn child. It touches deep-rooted fears relating to mental
incapacity, and above all it is surrounded with uncertainty – the
diagnosis may be in doubt for some weeks or even months, and the
prognosis is often extremely, and in the event often unnecessarily,
gloomy. The fears and anxieties dormant in all prospective parents
have suddenly been seen to have foundation.

'When she was born it was like a dream – I never knew anything about this, I didn't realise there was so much illness and handicap in the world, I was a person that was free. It was a shock' (Spain and Wigley, 1975).

Reaction

The shock may generate intense feelings of grief, anger, or despair; of a need to protect, coupled with the hope that the child will not survive; of bitterness at what life has brought and overwhelming feelings of inadequacy. It is unfortunate that many of the professionals involved initially often do not know how to react, so that a wall of silence grows. 'Health visitors . . . are not prepared for dealing with the birth of a handicapped child. They say a birth should be a joyous occasion – but they come in and find the parents stunned' (Simson, 1978). Parents need a sensitive and understanding response from the professional. They need an acceptance of their baby and of their own deep feelings, some of which cannot be acknowledged. They also need someone to talk to – 'I couldn't talk to my husband because he was upset too. My mother was shattered, I needed a stranger . . . .' (Bromley parent).

Most parents wish to be told the truth about the handicap of their child, and what they can expect in the future. Parents are only human and tend to hear what they want to believe. Information may therefore need to be repeated many times before the full implications are understood or accepted. Parents of mentally handicapped children frequently accuse doctors of withholding information, and while this is no doubt true in some cases, it does reflect a failure to realize both the extent of parental ignorance and the effects of the shock which makes it difficult for parents to absorb even the simplest information, particularly if it involves acceptance of reality. 'It is not a case of not knowing the answers, but of not even knowing the questions to ask' (McCormack, 1978).

A mother who had received a letter from a paediatrician stating quite specifically the nature of her child's disability could still tell her social worker five years later that nobody would tell her what was wrong. 'Somehow you just hope that something marvellous will happen; that some miracle will make it all right' *Newham Express* (1970).

Counselling

The need for counselling does not end with acknowledgement of the handicap. New situations will need to be faced, the marital relationship may be under stress, grandparents may refuse to accept the position, neighbours may show fear or lack of understanding. Above all parents will need help in working through their emotions. It is more comforting to seize on the inadequacies of the professionals involved, and blame them for their failures, than to face up to the devastating reality. The intensity with which parents will recall, many years later, the early months and the shortcomings of those who were in business to help them, is an indicator of the pain and stress which were undergone at the time.

Mourning

It is important to help parents and relatives mourn the child that might have been. 'Nothing can compensate for the loss of a normal daughter' (Hamilton, 1978); – 'It's worse than being bereaved' (Bromley parent); – 'You've just got to accept them for what they are and not keep wishing they were something else; not keep wishing they were normal' (Bayley, 1973). Eventually many families will be aware of the joy which a handicapped child often creates around him or her, and of how much they have learned in tolerance and understanding; but in the early months and years they need to be able to mourn the son who will never follow in father's footsteps, or the daughter who will never marry or have children of her own.

Fathers

The outward manifestation of the deep maternal feelings which develop in response to the awareness of handicap shows in a fierce protective attitude which tries to shelter the child from the world and everything in it. 'Any incident concerning her touched on emotional strings so deep that they vibrated at the slightest touch' (Collins and Collins, 1976).

In fighting the instinct not to reject that which is not perfect, the mother may put all her energies into caring for the child, to the detriment of her husband and other children. She may unconsciously blame the father, and in so doing refuse him opportunities to play a meaningful part in the physical caring and loving. 'I think more about him than about my husband because I think he needs more looking after than my husband' (Bayley, 1973). Fathers do not find it easy to talk out their feelings, nor does society offer many opportunities. Professional help, too, may only be on hand during the day.

Brothers and Sisters

It is very easy for the extraordinary care required by a mentally handicapped child to so occupy the parents' time that they have hardly a moment, or energy, to meet the emotional needs of any other children. Feeding problems, toileting, hyperactivity, sleeplessness – any or more of these may so distract the parents, and wear them down, that the other children are as shadows and their needs subordinated to those of their handicapped brother or sister. The preoccupation of the parents' thoughts and conversation with the progress and development of the handicapped child will start in the early months, and may continue as long as the handicapped child remains at home – to the exclusion of the achievements and milestones of the other children. The other children may feel their value is measured solely in relation to their response to the handicapped brother or sister, and their own feelings of guilt may be enhanced as they experience fluctuating feelings of love and hate. 'If Peggy had been an only child we could have justified all the extra time and trouble spent on bringing her up, but, looking back, I think we developed tunnel vision where this child was concerned and made mistakes because our view was so distorted' (Oswin, 1978).

Practical Help

If the family is to cope with the problem, and develop normally, it is vital that practical help is available. The usual situation is that neither parents, nor grandparents, nor friends, nor neighbours, have any experience or knowledge about mental handicap and the kind of services which are available. This places a tremendous responsibility on the professionals in touch with the family, to ensure that they are properly informed about what services are available, and that they know how to tap these services. In the infant years, coping with each stage of development, with behaviour difficulties and with relationships between siblings, may be the major preoccupation of the parents, particularly of the mother. 'The parents of a handicapped child are perpetually torn between the welfare of the handicapped child and keeping the rest of the family life as normal as possible' (Bromley Society, 1975). It is important to recognize the need for practical help regarding these day-to-day matters. Too often the professionals actually in touch with the family are not able to give this kind of help, but they should quickly recognize what is needed and call in other appropriate help. For instance, one mother found that her days were dominated by the trauma of meal-times when her handicapped daughter would regularly gain attention by throwing her food on the floor or at the wall, and this would be eagerly copied by her brother and sister. Any attempt to restrain her would bring on a temper tantrum which would further disrupt the meal, while attempts to rebuke the other children would be seen by them as completely unfair. Some advice from a psychologist concerning behaviour-modification would have made all the difference to this family.

Appropriate Advice

Advice given by professionals should recognize the need of parents to do something practical to help their handicapped child in the same way as they are able to help their other children. It should also recognize the nature of the family environment in which the child is living, and should be aimed at strengthening the coping mechanisms of the family. For example, it was of little use for one psychologist to recommend seclusion in a quiet room with his mother, for an hour at a time, as a solution to modify the hyperactive behaviour of a handicapped boy, when she had two other young children at home requiring care and attention.

Information

Most parents have an almost unassuageable thirst for information.

Starting in most cases from a state of complete ignorance they will seek information about all or any aspects of mental handicap, often in considerable detail; about the diagnosis, often showing dissatisfaction if a label cannot be attached to the handicap; about the prognosis, showing suspicion if this is uncertain about the future. Their ignorance may result in omission in their requests for information, and the professional needs to be alerted to this. For instance, parents are often completely unaware that there are any support services at all; therefore they need to have their attention drawn to these facilities.

Support Services

The mere provision of support services is not enough; it must be possible for the family to use a service without putting more strain on themselves by doing so. For example, a regular service such as a playgroup needs to offer transport, for even if the mother drives a car she may find that the effort of taking and fetching the child outweighs the advantage of the two hours or so she may have free. A babysitting service will fail if it does not put potential babysitters in touch with the families they are to help before they are needed, because the parents will be reluctant to leave their children with a stranger.

A support service must also be offered uncritically. A mother whose anxiety expresses itself in constant telephone calls to assure herself that her child is all right needs to be accepted on these terms and not as a nuisance, if she is to be able to use and benefit from the help which is available.

One of the most valuable support services can be provided by a short-stay unit if parents' needs are properly understood. A bureaucractic system which takes several weeks to process an application is not likely to be of much help in meeting short-term needs other than for the annual holiday, and therefore will lose much of its value. The quality of care must be good, and the child must be well treated – 'He came back just like a frightened animal. . . . It wasn't a bit of good, we went away and I had him on my mind all the time. When he came out he had bedsores and had lost half a stone in weight (Bayley, 1973). Some of the parents most in need of the unit may find it difficult to see it positively, as a means of keeping the family together, but see it only negatively, as a hidden rejection of the handicapped child. Any difficulty in obtaining the service will encourage them to continue to manage without; whereas help and support at an early stage could enable them to develop a pattern of use for the benefit of all the family.

All families are different, with enormous differences in their capacities to cope. Therefore it is essential that a range of support services should be available, and that every family should be aware of them and of how to benefit from them. Professional helpers tend to tell parents only about their own services, so that the parent-to-parent contact may be the major link in the information chain.

Contact with other Parents

In most areas there is a local group of parents (affiliated to a voluntary society such as the National Society for Mentally Handicapped Children) and most groups have a network of welfare visitors who provide support to parents in their neighbourhood. They give information on local services and have good links with local professional helpers. They can provide the individual contact for new parents, and support them until they feel ready to face other parents and to acknowledge the existence of other handicapped children. Other parents can help to break down the defensive barriers erected so hastily against the world, and while not denying the special nature of the new baby, can demonstrate the wealth of knowledge, experience and acceptance which can be gained from knowing others 'in the same boat'.

THE EARLY SCHOOL YEARS

'The Education Committee have carefully considered the advice which they have received from the Borough Medical Officer of Health as a result of your son's recent examination and all other information about J, and as a result they have decided that J is suffering from a disability of mind which makes him unsuitable for education at school and they propose to record this decision. After that the Committee will not be able to admit your son to any of their schools . . .' (Letter from Chief Education Officer of London Borough of Bromley; 2 August 1966).

209

For 15 years parents fought for legislation which would transfer responsibility for the education of all handicapped children from the local health authority to the local education authority, and in 1971 they succeeded – and the result has been dramatic.

So it may seem unreasonable to many teachers that parents do not just accept uncritically the resources offered by the local education authority, but often fail to respond to the help offered by the school, or respond in an aggressive and apparently hostile fashion. The generally beneficial effects on the child may be counterbalanced by considerable pressure on the family, depending on the effect of a number of factors:

The 3-Term Year

'I am convinced that school holidays often prove the final straw that makes parents give up on their good intentions and ask for hospital care' (McCormack, 1978). It is sometimes difficult for teachers, who feel they have borne the brunt during term time, to appreciate just how much mothers can dread the school holidays. Not only does the mother have to give over all her time to domestic tasks, she may also have to cope with behaviour difficulties and, as the children grow, so their diverging abilities make it increasingly difficult to organize activities which satisfy everyone.

For the mother with a child at boarding school, the relief afforded during term-time is no preparation for coping during the holidays, and in fact because of the re-assertion of normal life in the meantime, may make adjustment to what feels like the old crisis situation very difficult. The practical problems are intensified by emotional anguish, which re-lives, each holiday, the guilt and distress of what may appear to the parents as making the handicapped child pay the full penalty for their failure to cope – by being sent away.

Expectations

Perhaps the most important thing the educationists have brought to families is hope. The developmental approach enables teachers to build on each small step forward and to assess performance and devise individual learning programmes. Not only do parents have an important part to play in this; the very hope generated by the 'developmental model' leads parents to take an intensive interest in every sign of progress – and to become intensely concerned at what may appear a lack of it. Where relationships are positive, and communication good, the tension between teachers (whose expectations may at times be too low), and parents (whose expectations may be too high) can be healthy and work to the benefit of the child. Where the relationship is poor it can lead to frustration, conflict and bitterness, and increase the parents' feelings that the child is being offered a second-class service.

Communication between Home and School

Not every parent has had a good school experience, and their feelings towards the teachers and the school may be extremely ambivalent. This may make it difficult for parents to take the initiative in approaching the school when they are worried, or have the opposite effect of leading them to take an aggressive attitude which puts the teachers on the defensive.

Many schools have responded positively to the challenge and, faced by parents who have failed to find support and guidance from other services, have experimented with new ways of communicating on a level different from the daily written comments in the child's notebook. These experiments often involve groupwork such as parents' workshops, but in a situation where the school needs to sustain a good relationship for 11 years or more, it requires considerable skill on the part of the workshop or group leader to know where to draw the lines. As parents grow in confidence they may resent the intimate knowledge of their family/marital life which may have emerged in the group, and respond by distancing themselves from the teaching staff in an attempt to be viewed as 'normal' rather than as 'problems'. The opportunity for using a professional as a scapegoat for the parents' own failures or difficulties in coping may be beneficial if the relatively detached social worker is the target, but a stumbling block to greater understanding if the teacher is involved.

Transport

Life for many mothers can be haunted during term-time by

211

transport problems. Relief from the all-day caring of the infant years may be more apparent than real if it is substituted by a near-impossible timetable for the mother, in reconciling the pick-up and return-home times of the special-school minibus with the delivery and collection times of her children at other schools. The role of the escort, too, is crucial. Escorts are not usually trained, or even given induction training, but just pitchforked into the job. It is often mere chance which provides an escort who understands the pressures on the mother who has to meet the bus timetable, and at the same time who shows a warmth and tolerance towards the children.

Information

The need for information continues, but is likely at this stage to be focused on such matters as aspects of child development, how to complement the work of the school by teaching at home, the availability of welfare services, information about holidays, problems with brothers and sisters. Some parents will also wish to understand how the educational structure works and to know about the full range of educational facilities, not just the name of the nearest special school. Answers will be sought from anyone with whom the parents feel a rapport, and this may as often be other parents as professionals. Lack of knowledge should be frankly admitted, but help should be offered by suggesting other sources.

Contact with Other Parents

Many parents may shy away from contact with other parents, and find that to focus on the school is more comforting and a distraction from uncomfortable thoughts about the future. Where head teachers and staff are aware of the value of involving parents, a fruitful supportive relationship can develop which makes the school years something of an oasis. This, however, is more likely to happen if parents, too, understand where to draw the line, and do not expect teaching staff to provide the kind of mutual aid and willingness to see only the parents' point of view which can usually be obtained from other parents. As a final criterion, the teacher's first task is to educate the child. The secondary task is to share with others in supporting the family.

THE TEENAGE YEARS

'For all of us, the secret aspirations we might have had in our child's early years have had to change as the reality of the true pattern of development has been forced upon us' (Collins and Collins, 1976).

The Needs of the Mother

As the mentally handicapped child approaches the teens, a kind of depression may settle on the parents as a number of unacceptable options seem to lie ahead.

The hopes and aspirations of the early school years may be unfulfilled, and there looms ahead the adult training centre which may seem dull, unimaginative and repetitive by comparison with the school. Worse still, where there are insufficient adult centre places, the remaining school years are overshadowed, particularly for the mother, by the worry about what care will be provided and how soon, and just how long she is going to be able to cope. This may also be coupled with unexpressed feelings of resentment – just as she has begun to develop her own interests and social contacts, or even to undertake paid employment, she is now faced with a return to the restrictions of earlier years. She has watched many neighbours and friends resume old careers, or launch into new ones, and although she may not have been able to follow all the way, she may have been able to undertake a part-time paid or voluntary occupation which keeps her in touch with the outside world. In spite of the changing position of women in society as a whole, she may be faced with the fact that her position in the home is relatively unchanged, and it will be assumed that she alone amongst the members of the family will be expected, by relatives and professionals alike, to sacrifice her own aspirations and pick up the burden of care once more.

The Needs of the Family

The difficulties of coping with aggressive or overactive behaviour, running away, frustration, may be increasing as the child takes on the physical strength of an adult, and absorbs much of the parents' time and attention. 'The parents of a mentally handicapped child

213

are perpetually torn between the welfare of the handicapped child and keeping the rest of the family life as normal as possible' (Bromley Society, 1975), and keeping the balance can become increasingly difficult as brothers and sisters begin to develop distinctive individual identities and life-styles. Their tolerance may noticeably diminish if they are restricted in their opportunities to develop their own interests, or if space limitations in the home make it difficult to give them sufficient privacy. They may be embarrassed to bring their friends home, and may begin to grow accustomed to spending all their leisure time outside the home.

Coping with Puberty

'Every human being has the right to love and be loved, to establish a warm human relationship with someone of the opposite, or maybe the same sex. . . .' (Fairbrother, 1977).

All parents are threatened by the burgeoning and vigorous sexuality of their teenagers, and endeavour to cope with this by varying means of control. Through constant challenge, our normal sons and daughters ensure that these boundaries of parental control are continually widened – not always with parental support – until they gain full control over their own lives. This challenge cannot be presented by the mentally handicapped, and therefore their parents' acceptance of their maturity may be considerably delayed and, in many instances, never take place. The physical evidence of maturity may conflict with the parents' emotional response to the son or daughter as a child. It is very much harder to accept physical maturity to the full, and begin to reduce the level of supervision and to allow more freedom of choice. It is much easier to see the intellectual limitations and need for lifelong protection as a reason for continuing to exercise the detailed supervision of all aspects of life which were appropriate during earlier years.

The first manifestations of puberty are more likely to be behavioural than sexual. Normal adolescent behaviour may frequently be presented as abnormal in relation to the expectations of society, and the handicapped adolescent is not excluded from the enormous changes between the easy-going, happy, enthusiastic behaviour of many 11-year-olds and the bizarre, aggressive, apathetic, volatile behaviour of many adolescents. For parents, there is the same strain of coping and tolerating, and the same anxiety of wondering whether it really is just a passing phase or is the forerunner of what can be expected in the future, but intensified by the knowledge that the son or daughter will always be their responsibility. Added to this is the increase in physical conditions, like epilepsy, which frequently becomes more severe as the body undergoes the dramatic physical changes associated with puberty. As fits increase in number, the parents may find themselves covertly watching and waiting for the next one, so that at a time when the child is unconsciously seeking less oversight, he/she may in fact be receiving more.

Information – About Puberty

Parents who are involved in self-help groups are able to draw on each other's experience in handling the stage of puberty; others may turn to the schools, as few will be in touch with social workers, and doctors may be seen as too busy to spare the time; others may just rely on experience gained with their other children. Sex education is now considered an essential element in the secondary-school curriculum in order to help pupils learn to understand their emotions and developing sexuality, and how to function as adults. With the mentally handicapped, this help is needed by the parents. Professionals can provide positive support and information, often through the parents' workshops which have been developed in some areas.

Information – About the Future

Parents will need to learn about a different range of services, such as adult training centres or sheltered workshops; about adult education facilities; about different sources of advice and training such as disablement resettlement officers (DROs) and instructors. They will need guidance in knowing which of the many agencies involved is the appropriate one to approach. They will be confused at the multiplicity of professional help available, yet frustrated by its limitations. They will be unprepared for bureaucratic delays and procedures, and will tend to be both critical and hostile when they experience them for the first time. Not only, therefore, is it information that is required, but also guidance on how the system works, and the building-up of confidence to try to work it for themselves. For instance, it is not much help suggesting that contact be made with the social worker or DRO – what is needed is for the actual name, address and telephone number of each professional to be given, together with a description of their job, so that parents understand what they may reasonably expect that person to do.

Opportunities for Leisure

Opportunities to develop hobbies and recreational activities, and to go on holiday, temporarily freed from the responsibility of 24-hour caring, are important if parents are to be able to keep going year after year. But they will only feel free to enjoy themselves if there are also opportunities for the handicapped. So Gateway Clubs for young people, recreational classes, short-stay facilities and special holidays are essential if parents are to feel free to take a break from time to time to rest and relax and to play a favourite, sport or develop a hobby.

SPECIAL NEEDS

The Multiply Handicapped

Parents of the multiply handicapped have additional needs which call for special attention from the health service and social services. No longer will parents automatically accept that their children are 'hospital cases'. Many pride themselves on maintaining a normal family life for even the most profoundly handicapped, but they need help to cope with such problems as incontinence and physical management, which become more acute as childhood is left behind. A programme of daily care, to deal with incontinence and maintain standards of hygiene, needs to be developed. Also problems of lifting, which increasing weight and size generate, need to be solved if care is to be continued at home. 'Well it's that bath. Myself I think if there were a home help, even if it were only once a week, to come to assist with those main things . . .' (Bayley, 1973).

216

Incontinence aids, assistance with laundry, special clothing, hoists, bath aids and adaptations to the home, all assist parents to keep their son or daughter at home for as long as possible. Information about allowances is also important, as the extra costs involved – special diets, incontinence pads, extra heating, transport – can make it very difficult to manage on modest incomes. 'We just manage, we've got to be careful. Fuel is my big worry in winter . . .' (Bayley, 1973).

In particular it is important that the implications of the parents' decision to look after their son or daughter themselves are understood and accepted, so that on the one hand every effort is made to provide the basic services they need, and on the other they are not subjected to frequent pressure to agree to admission to hospital.

The Mildly Handicapped

The worries of parents with a mildly handicapped teenager may be particularly acute. Recognition of handicap may have been long delayed and only brought to light when the child shows difficulty in keeping up at school. But with good schooling, their sons and daughters may eventually be able to lead relatively normal lives, yet require someone in support to help when difficulties arise.

Jobs in open employment are not beyond the ability of these youngsters, yet recent changes in the employment market, which have reduced the supply of jobs suitable for the less able, may bring to nought the efforts of school and home to prepare them for the world of work, and force parents to consider facilities for sheltered employment.

Sexual maturity, too, brings worries of a different order. Young people able to develop a loving relationship may not easily understand the social norms related to premarital sex, nor the responsibilities involved in marriage and setting up their own home. Where residential support is needed, such facilities as exist may be geared to the severely handicapped when what is needed for the mildly handicapped is a group home or sheltered housing with help available when needed.

The loneliness of some mildly handicapped youngsters also

217

worries parents. The large catchment area of the special school may mean that friends live a long way away. Other young people may not be very tolerant, or may tend to exploit the slower person. In some areas clubs have been developed by parents specially for these youngsters to meet some of their social needs.

Overall the parents' underlying concern is enhanced by the vulnerability of their son or daughter. Intellectual limitations are often not visible, and outward appearances may not indicate the necessity for supervision and sometimes even protection.

THE ADULT YEARS

'I worry about the future. I didn't feel so much despair when I was young. It's grown since I've got older.' (Sinson, 1978).

Official Neglect

Older parents, with a mentally handicapped son or daughter living at home, are probably the most neglected in terms of support and help from both voluntary and statutory agencies. Considerable attention is given to the needs of parents and families in the early years, and the school provides a continuity of support from the age of 5, but the tendency to concentrate health and social service resources on acute situations provides little support for parents coping with the endless vista of adulthood. 'The thing is we just don't get any life, it's just the same thing over and over again, year in and year out' (Bayley, 1973). Where both parents are still involved, they may have built for themselves a way of life centred around the activities of their handicapped son or daughter which gives them opportunities for social contact, usually with other parents. Active help in the parent/teachers' association may have given way to support for the Gateway Club. The involvement of both partners also allows for the development of individual interests, although will not make it possible to develop joint activities. 'We don't go out together, we haven't done for years. . . .' (Bayley, 1973).

Coping Alone

Marriages weakened by the stress of earlier years may not withstand the prospect of unending restriction which lies ahead, or husbands may predecease their wives, so that mothers are frequently left solely responsible for the care of the handicapped adult. In addition to having to cope on their own, such mothers may be on low incomes and without transport, unable to envisage a life on their own, yet finding the physical burden of caring growing heavier all the time. In the case of boys additional problems may be presented by their growing physical strength.

The informal companionship of other parents, which may have been a great support in earlier years, may now be restricted as the opportunity to work and develop new interests takes other mothers away from the neighbourhood during the day, so that the isolation of those left behind is even more marked. The help which was once available from other sons and daughters will certainly have diminished as they take jobs, marry and develop family responsibilities of their own, so that the mother is left with a double burden – caring alone for her handicapped son or daughter, and coping alone with personal difficulties associated with ageing and poor health. 'I have my ups and downs actually, depending on Evelyn. One day I feel fairly well and another day, when Evelyn has been showing off, my nerves get topside of me' (Bayley, 1973).

Facing Reality

This is a time above all when it is no longer possible to avoid reality; acknowledgement has to be made that the son or daughter will never have a career, change jobs, experiment with different life-styles, or generally be drawn into the mainstream of human activity associated with work and leisure. Although attendance at an adult training centre may have removed some worries, such as how to cope in the school holidays, it may have resurrected feelings of anger and guilt if it is only offering a dull, unimaginative programme with undue attention being given to the performance of boring and repetitive industrial work at the expense of creative and educational activities. Years of fighting and pressing for services – 'Like almost everything else in the field of mental handicap, there are no spontaneous offers; everything has to be asked for' (McCormack, 1978) – coupled with a feeling that nothing they do will effect change, may induce an apathetic acceptance of the inevitable in parents' own responses.

A few may still have retained their vision and sufficient confidence in the future to seek to influence service-providers and/or to initiate provision themselves, but others may derive comfort from unrealistic expectations relating to employment in spite of all the evidence.

Is Help Acceptable?

Parents whose children are in their late twenties and older had to bring them up at a time when little help was available and they were compelled to cope on their own. Not only may they suffer from as serious a lack of information about available help as the young parents, but they may have very real difficulties in accepting help, partly because the relationship between the mother and handicapped child tends to be specially close when there is no husband. 'Well she is a companion for me and I don't know what I would do without her' (Bayley, 1973).

Anxiety, depression and frustration may show themselves in parents' continual expressions of criticism and discontent with whatever is offered. 'Officials must realise that they are often dealing with parents who are at the end of their tether, and who have had all their enthusiasm knocked out of them over the years' (Bromley parent, 1975).

This state of affairs is exacerbated by deep-rooted fears of the future which are difficult to acknowledge and, in contemplating residential care, the parents may be compelled to face up to a situation where the lynch-pin around which their lives have been structured is removed. 'He is depending on my life. I am only living for him' (Bayley, 1973).

RESIDENTIAL CARE

One thing I can say with confidence. Deciding to send your child to a residential school does not mean that you want to get rid of him. On the contrary, it can be the greatest demonstration of love that you can make' (Hamilton, 1978).

Is Home the Right Place?

To those observing the difficult situation of families trying to cope, for example, with an overactive child, the obvious answer may be to find a residential place. To the parents the position may be quite different. Of course, there are instances of rejection and/or abuse, when the child needs to be taken away for its own protection; but to the majority of parents, home is the right place for all their children to live.

It is not an easy matter for a mother to accept the need for help or to admit she is unable to cope. 'Never have I got over the feeling of not being able to cope. Every visit to the hospital has been a reminder that I am inadequate' (McCormack, 1978).

There is also the mother's guilt as she feels she is contemplating the action because of her own needs rather than the child's. 'If he did go away I'd have a lot more freedom than I do now; that's why I want him to go; therefore, it's wrong for him to go' (Hamilton, 1978).

The father may be torn between his devotion to the handicapped child and his inability to give his wife the support and help she needs during the day, or even to cope himself when he is at home, which makes it almost impossible to contemplate sending away the most vulnerable member of the family.

The whole process of educating the public to accept the right of the mentally handicapped to as normal a life as possible, also puts pressure on the parents to resist all thoughts of residential care, which is seen as a regressive move with connotations of the bad old days.

Because every family is different, and what one family can cope with brings another to breaking point, parents who have learned to appreciate and rely on the support of other parents may find that in this one crucial matter they are on their own.

'It takes tremendous determination to make the decision to send your child away, however much it may benefit the family as a whole and even if it has been recommended by the professional involved with the child. You have to be prepared to do battle with the authorities, fifty per cent of interested bystanders (the other half are pushing you in various other directions) and your conscience' (McCormack, 1978).

Information

No decision can be made in a vacuum, and as part of the process of deciding whether or not to seek residential care for their child, parents will need to learn about the kind of residential facilities which exist, and what is available to them in terms of care; the policy of the local authority regarding financial support; eligibility; length of waiting lists. The shortage of places and financial restrictions may tend to make this information hard to come by, as local authorities tend to discourage requests for residential provision.

Facts alone are not what is needed. Parents also need to see schools, homes, or hospitals for themselves, to meet some of the staff, and to learn about their philosophies and aims. So guidance on how to arrange visits, and dates of open days, should be given.

Seeking a Place

Once a decision to seek residential help has been made, there may follow a long, tortuous period while a place is sought. The policy of local authorities varies enormously – from supporting the parents' decision, and doing all in their power to find a suitable place, to resisting any consideration of help until a crisis is reached. Too often, in spite of the continual strain they are under, the parents themselves are left to find a place. If the parents are not united in their decision, delay may increase the tension between them. Indeed the very act of contemplating relief from ongoing strain may make it hard to cope until a firm date for admission has been received.

Learning to Live with It

The special agony of these families intensifies when the child eventually leaves. The relief from an intolerable burden can but increase the mother's feelings of guilt, unless she is helped to understand her feelings. Bewildered brothers and sisters, equally relieved at the relaxing of domestic tension, may feel guilt and responsibility as unspoken wishes seem to have come true, or, if too young to understand the reasons, may show a great deal of insecurity. The parents may feel rejected by those from whom they would normally expect to turn for understanding, by the staff in whose care the child has been placed, and by other parents. The parents' need to continue to play a part in the caring and decision-making relating to the handicapped child may be ignored. Even the relief may only be temporary, as each year is punctuated by school holidays which may re-create the very situation which determined the need for residential care in the first place; in this situation there is rarely any help at hand.

Fear of the Future

For older parents, fear of the future is all-pervading but almost too dreadful to contemplate. 'I realise how wrong it is but one wishes that we could take her with us when we die. I find I cannot think about any sort of thing. Her death seems much easier to contemplate. I know it's wrong but there you are' (CARE, 1971). Many parents will not consider their possible need for long-term care when the kind of residential care they want for their child is not available. It is not surprising that in one survey only 21% of the parents would consider the possibility of care before it became inevitable, when the kind of residential care desired bore no relation to the type of residential care currently available (Bromley Society, 1975). Professionals know that in an emergency the social services will move in and make appropriate arrangements, but many parents are unaware of this fact. 'It's desperate – no one will care for him. Perhaps someone from the Society [for Mentally Handicapped Children] will visit him. He is not seen as handicapped, just a menace to society' (Bromley parent, 1975).

It is the little things that worry parents, the simple facts of everyday home life that can get overlooked in an institution: 'I worry about silly things, petty little things. Will they wipe her nose when she has a cold? Will they wipe her bottom? If she bumps her head, will they kiss her? She always comes to me for a kiss when she hurts herself and that makes it better. I just hope they will look after her the way we do. If we could be sure S— was happy, it would go a long way towards making us happy' (McCormack, 1978).

The Mildly Handicapped

For parents of the more mildly handicapped, the situation is particularly grim because there are few suitable places available.

At least with the severely subnormal there can be no question that continuing care is needed; but the paradox of the less handicapped may lie in their ability to take a job in open employment but not to take full responsibility for every aspect of their lives. Places in subnormality hospitals and hostels, where they exist, may be totally unsuitable for the individual who can live in some degree of independence provided there is some oversight and overall care. For these parents contemplation of the future may be unbearable unless they can engage in a joint initiative to create a group home or sheltered housing scheme.

SUMMARY

Parents are rarely prepared for the birth of a mentally handicapped child. Families rarely contain within their ranks the experience which will help the parents to cope. Parents, relatives and friends rarely have information on services available or knowledge of where to go for it.

It is important, therefore, that community services which are developed to meet the needs of the mentally handicapped, should also take the needs of parents and families into account. Above all, it is essential that they should be based on the availability of life-long support.

Support by Professionals

In Adjustment

Parents require support during the process of adjustment, but it needs to be recognized that this is not confined to the early months and years. Parents have to adjust to each stage of development right into adulthood, for there is no such thing as complete acceptance. A particularly difficult time is in the early teens; while coming to accept the implications of mental handicap in adulthood can be exceedingly stressful.

In Understanding

There is a need for professionals to understand the depth of feeling involved at all stages and to accept, as normal, feelings which

might be seen by the parents either to be abnormal, or too unacceptable to express even to themselves. In the early days
particularly, parents will be looking for a magic formula, rather
than seeking ways in which they can cope. When the professional is
unable to produce this formula, the parents will initially find
comfort in reacting aggressively, rather than in facing up to the
reality of a long-term situation. 'At . . . times, anger, hostility,
resentment and criticism may call for support of a psycho-
therapeutic nature' (King's Fund Centre, 1976). There is a need to
recognize that, as with all people there is infinite variety amongst
parents in their response to a situation and their ability to cope.
There is no one answer.

As Partners

'The parents' role is not fixed; it may change from time to time,
varying from dependence to co-partnership, and on to leadership
at times' (King's Fund Centre, 1976). The report of a group of
parents and professionals, meeting under the auspices of the King's
Fund Centre, identified the need for professionals to recognize
parents as 'co-partners in a difficult enterprise'. Professional
expertise can back up and reinforce the parents' instincts and
convictions about what is right for their child, but in a complex life-
long situation, where there is no one 'right' answer, it is only in a
spirit of partnership that the parents will feel supported, and
service to the child be maintained.

This requires recognition of the parents' changing role but 'if a
basis of co-partnership has been developed early in the life of the
handicapped person, it is likely to persist, even though occasionally interspersed by periods of much greater dependence' (King's
Fund Centre, 1976).

With Honesty

'Absolute honesty by the professional is essential' (King's Fund
Centre, 1971).
Firstly, in relation to the practical problems of caring at home:
  '. . . admitting that the situation is difficult or the outlook
  gloomy, is a far cry from saying flatly, or even implying, that

225

there is nothing more to be done. For who knows if this is so, in a field of work so full of surprises? Certainly it is wrong to give false hope, but it is equally wrong to destroy hope. Parents must have hope, not for a wonder cure, but the chance that something more – however modest – may be done to alleviate the situation or prevent deterioration'.

Secondly, in relation to assessment: it is essential that parents are present and actively involved as equal partners in all case conferences and assessment procedures.

Thirdly, in relation to the sharing of information: it is still a highly contentious matter to promote the right of parents to see notes on official files about their child. Doctors, teachers, social workers, disablement resettlement officers, and many others, jealously guard the confidentiality of their notes. Yet 'parental involvement is impossible to visualize without sharing of information' (King's Fund Centre, 1976), and it is important that clear, written reports based on the working notes of professionals should be given to parents.

Support by other Parents

'A feeling by parents that with the best training and the best will in the world, professionals cannot really understand their child or their problems' (McCormack, 1978). There is no substitute for the support and understanding on many levels which can be derived from contact with other parents, and every encouragement, through the provision of appropriate information and/or personal introduction to other parents, needs to be given to help new parents form their first contact with others. This is not always easy to develop, requiring as it does acknowledgment that their own child is mentally handicapped and acceptance that, as parents, they are in the same situation as others. Parents of the mildly handicapped have particular difficulties here, but once contact is established, they too find infinite support at many levels in their association with other parents.

Acknowledgment

I am grateful for the advice received in the preparation of this chapter from a number of parents (members of the Bromley Society for Mentally Handicapped Children), some of whose comments have been quoted.

References

Bayley, M. (1973). *Mental Handicap and Community Care. A Study of Mentally Handicapped People in Sheffield.* (London: Routledge & Kegan Paul)

Bromley Society (1975). *A Life Apart. (A survey of the problems and needs of the mentally handicapped and their families in the London Borough of Bromley.)* (London: Bromley Society for Mentally Handicapped Children)

CARE (1971). *The Mental Health Explosion.* (Prepared and published by CARE for the Mentally Handicapped)

Collins, M. and Collins, D. (1976). *Kith and Kids. Self-help for Families of the Handicapped.* (London: Souvenir Press (E&A))

Day, K. A. (1977). Services for pre-school mentally handicapped children and their families. *GLAD News,* October

Fairbrother, Pauline (1977). Love and affection. *Health and Social Services Journal,* LXXXVII, no. 4570

Hamilton, J. (1978). Caring enough to let go. *Parents Voice,* 28, 3

Kings' Fund Centre (1976). *Collaboration between Parents and Professionals.* Mental Handicap Paper 9. (Kings' Fund Centre)

McCormack, M. (1978). *A Mentally Handicapped Child in the Family.* (London: Constable & Co.)

Newham Express (1970). 'The twilight world'. 23 January

Oswin, M. (1978). *Holes in the Welfare Net.* (London: Bedford Square Press)

Sinson, J. (1978). 'Charting success'. A Down's group in Leeds. *Nursing Times Community Outlook,* Vol. 14, no. 23

Spain, B. and Wigley, G. (1975). *Right from the Start. A Service for Families with a Young Handicapped Child* (NSMHC)

Suggested Additional Reading

Travelling Hopefully. (Greenwich Society for Mentally Handicapped Children)

Planning for the Future. (Renée Wheeler: Borough of Barnet Society for Mentally Handicapped Children, and NSMHC)

14

ASSISTING THE FAMILIES OF THE MENTALLY HANDICAPPED

E. Jones

The characteristic of the mentally handicapped which most concern parents and teachers, and which must be overcome, is the fact that the extent of their learning is not only limited but frequently, because of inadequate and insufficient teaching, what they do learn is inappropriate.

In the pre-school child, impairment of skills such as walking, talking, eating, toileting, undressing and dressing are the main areas in which impaired adaptive behaviour can be seen. For the school-age child the slow learning of academic skills becomes important, whereas for adults, the inability to function independently in the community or to maintain adequate behaviour in job performance singles them out. Tizard and Grad in 1959 wrote:

> No simple answer can be given to the question: What is it like to have a mentally subnormal child and what should one do about it? The children themselves differ greatly in degree of mental handicap, temperament, physical health and ease of management. Families differ also both in the number of other problems they have to cope with and in their ability to cope. The assistance given by health and welfare agencies varies in time and place and in quality.

PROBLEMS AND QUESTIONS

In setting out to help families make as rich and satisfying an experience as possible out of a very tough human situation it is important to define the areas in which you seek to be of service.

The White Paper (1971), 'Better Services for the Mentally Handicapped', states that 80% of handicapped children and 40% of mentally handicapped adults live at home. Among the problems and questions with which families are confronted are:

Acceptance of the handicapped child.
Why did this happen to us?
Will he ever be able to look after himself and, if not, who will do this when they are no longer able to do so?
Obtaining advice on management.
Can the family provide the care the child needs?
Will their child get any fun out of life?
Statutory benefits and allowances.
Is the accommodation adequate?
Opportunities for rest and leisure for themselves and the child.
What can we do for others?

There is no particular order to such questions; some persist, others recur; there is no simple answer to any of them. Some families cope very well and remain cohesive and creative units in which their children grow up normally and happily – others are overwhelmed by the handicapped child and eventually disintegrate.

ATTITUDES TO THE HANDICAPPED AND THEIR FAMILIES

Although there remains a great deal of prejudice from members of the public, usually from ignorance, attitudes towards handicapped people and their families have changed considerably over the last 25 years. The importance of the change is that it allows and enables new scope for the handicapped, their families and for those who seek to help them.

It is important to recall that it is only about 25 years ago that if parents had a severely handicapped child, then they were advised as part of the 'then' good practice to place their child in an institution. This remains within the memory of some citizens today. Many works from 1960 onwards showed that severely handicapped children brought up in their own homes and families were more forward in their development than those brought up in institutions. Thus, the previous over-evaluation of institutions and the over-optimistic view of what they were likely to achieve for their residents gave way to pressure on parents to keep the handicapped child at home, and to the policy which we now endorse of maintaining the mentally handicapped in the community as far as is practicable.

EFFECTS ON THE FAMILY

Let us consider what having a handicapped child means to a family.

A handicap that is present at birth or at an early age will interfere, at least initially, with the natural processes which enable parents to fall in love with their children. The word process is an important one, both from the point of view of the child and the parents. A man and woman adopt new roles when they become husband and wife and these roles again change when they become parents. There is a natural anxiety that occurs in all pregnancies and the first question so often is 'Is it all right?' or the kind midwife says so quickly 'a lovely boy, ten fingers and ten toes'. When the infant arrives in the family, he also plays a role and the early responses in the infant help to release the reciprocal responses in the mother; so commences an interaction between mother and child. At first the mother meets all the child's needs and gradually allows the outside world to come in. Mothers and fathers do this naturally, thus enabling development to take place, and by the age of 5 years the normal child has learnt many of the skills and responses necessary for an eventual adult existence. Indeed, in our society we expect children by the age of 5 years to be able to leave their homes, walk to school, cross the busy main road with the help of the 'lollipop lady', stay there during the day, sit, attend, comprehend, play, cope with their toileting and feeding during the day, as well as accept the formal educational system.

231

What happens when the child is handicapped? Imagine the child with Down's syndrome, spina bifida or early-diagnosed abnormality, such as phenylketonuria. Instead of the usual relief that all is well and that the baby is normal, the unexpected and unpleasant has occurred and the feeling is one of intense crisis; parents will speak of how they feel numb, disgusted, empty and helpless, how they just could not accept the fact, how they feel a sense of guilt and shame, of how they blame themselves and of the extreme anxiety they felt.

The expected perfect child has been lost and the feared damaged child has been born. At this time parents need help to work through the mourning for the loss of the normal child and help to accept the handicapped child. The initial diagnosis comes as a terrible shock and at this stage the family need considerable emotional support. They also need specific information with guidance towards available treatment, management and the future. At this stage the family, and the professionals who are going to help them, have to come to an agreement that there will be help throughout the life of the handicapped member. The nearer this comes to a contract between parents and professionals the better, with parents letting professionals know what their needs are and what they honestly expect, and professionals likewise honestly stating what they expect of parents and setting goals for the child. Parents and professionals need to agree as to what is realistic for the child and to review and alter goals in the light of what happens.

PROFESSIONALS INVOLVED

It is important to realize that professional workers also have to work through similar feelings of loss, grief and anger before they can be maximally effective in helping the handicapped child and the family.

The professionals move on, change jobs for experience or promotion, they may become ill themselves – all of this can impose a large number of professionals on the family with the handicapped member, and these changes can be seen as a loss also.

No one professional can give all the help required and it is necessary for the family to see that many professional people are showing their concern and using their skills to help the family. If repeated or prolonged hospitalization is necessary in the early period of the child's life, then this can increase the despair and rejection. Fears and anxiety for the present and the future have to be ventilated; guilt must be recognized and relieved but not over-inflated and wrongly used.

TELLING PARENTS

When do you tell parents of a handicap in their child? All the evidence points to the value of early diagnosis and to giving specific diagnostic information as soon as the mother is through the physiological shock of the birth process. The information given must be followed up by further support. Most parents prefer to be told early but it is important that they can come back with questions and anxieties as they need to. Undoubtedly, it is better to see mother and father together, as it is very wrong to let mother tell father, so causing her to answer his questions and face his hostilities, while at the same time cope with her own. One writer likened informing the parents to the performance of a surgical operation without an anaesthetic. It is important to share information about the handicap and to provide information about community and other resources during the initial introductory interviews. The giving of information is also a sharing of professional commitment to the family. Too often parents are said to be emotionally overwhelmed when, in fact, they are informatively deprived.

When do you tell the other children in the family about the new member's handicap? The concept of slowness and of slow learning needs to be communicated as soon as it can be grasped. At 9–10 years of age more specific details can be shared and from then onwards better understanding can continue.

INITIAL ACCEPTANCE BY THE FAMILY

The initial acceptance of the child is very important – this depends to a very large extent on how the parents themselves were treated as children. If, as a child, a parent was rejected or over-protected, then as an adult, that parent will be affected in terms of self-regard,

233

self-confidence and the ability to be a parent, all of which are influenced by handicap in the child.

Acceptance takes time – it involves a process, as the loss of the normal child must also be worked through. Parents require considerable support during this time – grandparents are often of little help as they too have to work through their own feelings which may be even stronger than those in the parents.

Helplessness in the newborn baby is normal but when this persists and the natural developmental milestones are not achieved, there is disappointment at each stage: the advances of the neighbour's child rub it in, developmental checks and clinics can also rub it in. At each stage there is a repeated feeling of loss, anger, depression and rejecting feelings; fear of abuse, anxiety, bodily aches and pains can all result.

On top of all this, there may be other problems – financial, housing, marital conflict, pressure from siblings, disturbed behaviour from siblings and a severe restriction of social life.

As parents we require a response from our children – a smile, the appropriate development of language or a social skill – the parent of a handicapped child can miss out on all these satisfactions. We also like our children to travel the journey towards independence – the parents of a handicapped child have to tolerate a prolonged dependency on themselves.

The grief and anger at the blow that life has dealt them are said to be almost universal reactions of the parents of the handicapped child, and before they are likely to accept the child's handicap they have to work through a series of different adjustment stages – the period of grief – then learn how to acknowledge and express their anger – then deal with the anxieties that the particular handicap arouses – then make adjustments in their way of life that will affect not only the handicapped child but the total family unit. The late Dr Mary Sheridan wrote in 1965: 'It is no exaggeration to say that in the background of every individual handicapped child there is always a handicapped family.' Indeed, professionals should always be aware of the whole family and not merely the handicapped member. We need to be concerned not only about the specific nature of the handicap and its problems but also the family dynamics, social, physical and educational needs of various members.

The family of the handicapped person can be said to experience a chronic sorrow which is a natural reaction to a tragic fact. The reality of handicap for the family is its presence in a loved one 24 hours a day, 7 days a week, 52 weeks a year.

The coping mechanisms chosen by a handicapped family will vary with that family's characteristics and resources and with the nature and degree of the stress.

FORECASTING THE FUTURE

To answer questions about the future development of the handicapped child can be very difficult. It is hard to find a balance between wanting to avoid being dogmatic and the wish to meet the parents' rightful need for information. The presence of previous non-handicapped children in the family is helpful in understanding normal development, while the work of Dr Sheridan is helpful to parents and professionals alike.

REACTIONS OF OTHER CHILDRĒN

Brothers and sisters are very important in the handicapped family. The handicap can result in the neglect of brothers and sisters, older and younger. They can be given increased responsibility for caring for the handicapped person, both in the present and projected into the future. On occasions they can displace their anger towards the handicapped person to acting out behaviour outside the home. They may be embarrassed by the stigma of handicap and show considerable anxiety in adolescence, before marriage or before childbearing. There is need to allow them to talk to others about their feelings and fears.

TELLING OTHER RELATIVES, NEIGHBOURS, FRIENDS AND ACQUAINTANCES

Connected to knowing about the handicap and accepting it is the question of being able to tell others that a family member is handicapped. To be able to say, 'Yes, this is my latest child, he has some kind of handicap.'

It is necessary to be able to present the child to the community. If a parent is unable to do so, this leads to social withdrawal for the parents and child and to other family members becoming ashamed of the handicapped person. Encouragement has to be given to parents to present the child in an open and honest way. For some, contact with other parents with a handicapped child is helpful; this must never be forced on parents but offered to them to freely use or refuse.

HELPING PARENTS TO BE INVOLVED IN DEVELOPMENT

The acquistion of social competence is of major importance in the developing child. The normal child acquires social skills through incidental learning in the course of growing up. The mentally handicapped child fails to acquire such information incidentally, gets it wrong and has to be formally taught these skills which will help him to get along and to conform to the minimum requirements for living in the community. Social competence is extremely important in the acceptance of the mentally handicapped person in the community. The normal average child is largely competent in these terms by the time he has to go to school. Some children acquire these skills quickly and easily while others are a lot slower and the normal variation is, in fact, very wide. A very important factor in the acquisition of these skills is the parental expectation of the child. The important social skills are: feeding oneself, toileting oneself, undressing and dressing appropriately, washing and the ability to play.

The acquisition of these skills is related to intelligence and in the handicapped slow-learning child it is necessary to offer specific training programmes to help the child acquire them. It is important to say to parents, 'You are a great mother/father, you have also to be a great teacher of your handicapped child.'

Let us focus briefly on dressing; undressing and dressing require a high degree of physical agility combined with sufficient perceptual maturation to be able to control the limbs and trunk in this skill and to be able to perceive shapes, sizes, colours and to be aware of one's own body in space.

The normal average child begins to co-operate with mother in dressing at 12–18 months; by 3 years such a child can pull down pants and at 5 years can undress and dress completely with the exception of difficult buttons or laces.

The mentally handicapped child has to be formally taught these skills, and certain habits, such as inappropriate undressing, persist longer. If advised correctly parents can be the most able teachers and can use the principles of learning theory to help their slow-learning child acquire skills. One very important aspect is that parents, like care staff, should use all the naturally occurring situations to teach, such as getting up, going to bed and mealtimes.

In teaching dressing skills the child not only learns to dress but to distinguish colours, clothes, size, style, as this is an exercise in perceptual training as well as in a social skill. The likelihood is that the handicapped child able to dress himself will be the handi-capped adult with sufficient perceptual skills to do simple assembly work.

In helping parents to help their handicapped child there is the acknowledgment that parents are the best teachers of their handi-capped child. Definitions of mental handicap put emphasis on the current behaviour of the handicapped person and view handi-capped behaviour as a failure of learning. Parents no longer accept traditional views such as subnormal mentality, and more and more want to be involved in helping their child learn and develop. Parents should be offered a service which allows early recognition of handicap and sets out as early as possible to teach new skills. It is wrong to wait until there is a problem. What we can be really good at together, parents and professionals, is in teaching new skills, dressing, feeding, comprehension, play and more complicated skills. We are relatively poor at dealing with problem behaviour or established wrong learning.

ESSENTIALS FOR PARENTS AND PROFESSIONALS WORKING TOGETHER

The essential implication of this is that we, parents and professionals, study and share the principles of how people learn, how new skills are taught and how we can learn to do the right thing in the right place. We need to study and share together how we set realistic goals and decide the most appropriate things to teach. We need to get together when we get it wrong and problem behaviour results. Within learning theory, developmental paediatrics and goal-setting we have worthwhile principles on which we can work together. At the end of the chapter reference is made to literature that will be helpful to study and share, for parents and professionals.

In conclusion, the following principles should not be forgotten by professionals who set out to help handicapped people and their families:

> be honest with parents, most of whom are not prepared to accept the platitudes frequently used to camouflage ignorance;
>
> do not take the problem over;
>
> help parents themselves to work at the changing developmental issues;
>
> you cannot generalize about handicapped children or their parents;
>
> watch your language when speaking to parents;
>
> parents of handicapped persons are also people like yourself;
>
> remember they are the parents of the child;
>
> no decision should be for ever, but re-evaluate and up-date in the light of new skills and resources.

I would also like to recognize that I exist professionally only as part of a team of people who share many skills together. The development of such teams working from community units is proving more and more rewarding both for parents and professionals.

I would like to express a very big 'Thank you' to all those parents of handicapped persons who have helped me to help them and theirs.

References and Further Reading

Better Services for the Mentally Handicapped. Cmnd 4683 (1971). London: HMSO)

Ehlers, W. H., Krishef, C. H. and Prothero, J. C. (1973). *An Introduction to Mental Retardation: A Programmed Test.* (USA: Charles E. Merril Publishing Co.)

Gordon, S. (1975). *Living Fully: A Guide for Young People with a Handicap, their Parents, their Teachers and their Professionals.* (USA: The John Day Co.)

Perkins, E. A., Taylor, P. D. and Capie, A. C. M. (1976). *Helping the Retarded: A Systematic Behavioural Approach.* (Kidderminster: British Institute of Mental Handicap)

Perske, R. (1973). *New Directions: For Parents of Persons who are Retarded.* (Nashville, USA: Co-operative Publication Association)

Sheridan, M. D. (1975). *Children's Developmental Progress, From Birth to Five Years.* (Windsor: NFER)

Tizard, J. and Grad, J. (1959). *The Mentally Handicapped and Their Families: a Social Survey.* (London: Oxford University Press)

15

PLAY, TOY LIBRARIES AND ADVENTURE PLAYGROUNDS

E. Jones

Many theories have been advanced to account for the value of play. This is not an occasion for a review of these theories but rather to advocate that play has a major place in the services that we provide for mentally handicapped children.

WHAT IS PLAY?

It is amazingly difficult to define play precisely, as the concept involves recreation, amusement, fun, merry-making, sport, comedy, tragedy, performance, freedom of movement, space and much much else. Essentially there is no one definition as there are as many different play behaviours as there are people engaged in those behaviours.

An important question often asked by the parents of a handicapped child is will their child get any fun out of life? Ability to play is also linked with the concept of happiness.

LEARNING PLAY

In recognizing a child to be handicapped it is important to also value that child and to put over to parents that their child, although handicapped, is still a very worthwhile person. It is important at a very early stage to give parents the perspective that children learn through play and that like any other skill play behaviour can be taught. A parent once said, 'You are the first person [professional] to say anything nice about him.' Another parent said, 'Before I went to the Toy Library I never thought of buying him toys to teach him anything.'

Many years ago, in a magazine called *Help,* I read a poem by Muriel, then aged 10 years – I have shared it with many people because of its developmental content:

> At the age of one you have just begun,
> At the age of two you are you,
> At the age of three you play in the sea,
> At the age of four you stand at the door.
> At the age of five you can survive,
> At the age of six you play tricks,
> At the age of seven you think of heaven,
> At the age of eight you swing on the gate,
> At the age of nine you are fine,·
> At the age of ten you change.

PLAY DEVELOPMENT

Indeed, in our society we expect a 5-year-old child to be able to leave mother and father, walk to school, sit, attend, comprehend, play, be competent in 'self-help' skills, share, be happy and return to his parents at the end of the day.

In working with parents, acknowledging the chronological age of their child, I often ask mother at what developmental level she would place her child. Parents are normally spot-on in answering this difficult question, which often helps them see their child's difficulty in a realistic way and allows an entry to setting a teaching target for parents.

A good deal is known and documented about normal development which is a continuous process from conception to maturity and depends primarily on the maturation of the nervous system. The sequence of development is the same in all children but the rate of development varies from child to child and is influenced by parental expectation.

The work of Sheridan, Gunzberg and Illingworth, and many other people, very usefully records time-scales and variations of development and these works are frequently referred to by all of us working with children. However, these various tables tend to be selective of a small number of skills and there is no one chart that covers development and most importantly tells us what the next teaching task should be.

So often we do not give play the respect that it deserves. The oft-heard expression 'He is only playing' strangely devalues behaviour that is even more important to the child than work is to the adult. Indeed as work skills become re-evaluated, as our technological achievements advance, we may all find ourselves seeking to learn play skills and having to produce more play behaviour than ever before.

An awareness of normal development and the assets, deficits and excesses of behaviour of the handicapped child clues us in to what we should be teaching in respect of play or any other skill. We can teach play skills as we teach any other skills.

THE SCOPE OF PLAY

Play allows children to enter the world that is theirs and ours where we share touch, sight, smell, shape, size, colour, movement of many kinds and complexity and the sounds of objects and voices. These perceptual exercises merge with success and failure, joy and frustration and allow more complex tasks to follow the earlier simpler learning that has emerged. Laughter, tears, anger and joy have their place, and various activities help the child work out his feelings about himself in relation to his world and his future. Each individual child will travel his own developmental journey according to his own road map. By valuing play we can maximize the journey that the child travels.

THE TOY LIBRARY AS A GUIDE TO PLAY

In 1972 the then Institute of Mental Subnormality (now British Institute of Mental Handicap) set up a Toy Library. The organization of a Toy Library is well-documented by Barbara Wroe in the BIMH publication *Organizing a Toy Library: A Description of the*

243

IMS Toy Library Service. this booklet outlines the main purposes of the Toy Library as:

1. To provide parents of handicapped children with advice and guidance on the importance of play and appropriate play materials, and to help them set realistic aims for their children to achieve.

2. To lend suitable toys and play equipment, cassette tapes (of short stories and nursery rhymes) and (in the case of the physically handicapped) instrumental aids for use at home and to guide the parents on how to use them most effectively in order to develop their child's skills.

3. To liaise closely with other people involved with 'the family', such as teachers, nurses, social workers, health visitors, speech therapists and physiotherapists and medical practitioners in the various disciplines concerned.

4. To provide information and advice to pre-school and nursery groups, special schools, hospital wards and other voluntary or official organizations intent on establishing their own libraries, on 'value for money' equipment and the ranges of items most suitable for their particular needs.

This booklet describes the necessary premises and equipment, the playroom and supporting facilities. It gives succinct details of how the library is organized in terms of information on play materials and how they can be obtained. It gives advice about buying toys, hints on their care and maintenance and the placement of toys in various categories which have different teaching value is explained. Over a period of time a record emerges of the toys, activities and learning tasks that apply to a particular child. In the time the library has functioned, we have valued the work of the librarians whose professional backgrounds have included mental handicap nursing, nursery nursing and teaching. The librarians have accepted referrals of a wide variety of professional people including:

Psychiatrists	Hospital nurses (mental handicap)
Health visitors	
Physiotherapists	Peripatetic teachers of the deaf
Teachers	Area medical officers of health
Paediatricians	Peripatetic teachers of the blind

Parents	Neurologists
Social workers	Playgroup leaders
Community nurses	Hospital medical officers
(mental handicap)	Speech therapists
Psychologists	

The booklet details the kind of information kept on a child and family, and gives an indication of the very wide variety of handicaps that have been seen.

The role of this Toy Library is inevitably influenced by conceptualizing handicap as a disorder of learning, and adopts a behavioural approach to the teaching of play skills. The publication *Helping the Retarded – a Systematic Behavioural Approach* by Perkins, Taylor and Capie is a helpful explanation of the approach and in particular the Developmental checklist of this publication is completed on each child, referred and up-dated at intervals to record the progress made by the child. Perkins and Taylor also wrote two articles called 'Learning Through Play', in *Apex* in 1976; these describe play in the context of normal development and in relation to the mentally handicapped child. The authors set out a useful play plan which deals with skills relevant to shape and sorting, building, manipulation, social games, gross motor activities and imaginative play. The articles detail the equipment necessary to the teaching tasks related to the above skills.

THE TOY LIBRARY AS A THERAPEUTIC ESSENTIAL

The aims of the Toy Library have been quoted, but much more happens. So often the Toy Library is seen by parents as a safe place, and the librarians as safe people with whom they feel quite able to share all kinds of fears and anxieties about their children. The librarians are free to visit homes, schools, or any place where they can share their skills with people concerned with and for the mentally handicapped. Many professionals are alerted to difficulties that they would not otherwise hear of, or hear of much later when nearer to crisis. Freedom of contact between the Toy Librarians and other professionals engaged in helping the handicapped child is encouraged.

ADVENTURE PLAYGROUNDS

Whereas mental handicap does limit the vocational and social functioning of the individual this is not nearly so much as is often assumed. All children require a place where they can play, find space and freedom to run about making a noise while investigating the world around them. If an environment can be produced which stimulates the children's imagination and challenges them to face and overcome risks, then this will help children build up self-confidence and independence.

Often the mentally handicapped are over-protected, told to take care, watched closely in case of danger. Like everyone else the handicapped person needs to learn courage with which to face life. There is something healthy in risk-taking and a crippling indignity in over-protection and over-stressed safety.

Apex, in June 1974 (vol. 2, no. 1), contained an article on the design and construction of an adventure playground at a hospital for the handicapped. It offers a child many different experiences – crawling through a tunnel, sliding, climbing a rope, crossing a bridge, a plank walk, sand and water play. It offers the dignity of risk in a reasonably challenging play environment that is within sensible adult concern. It expands the horizon of children whose lives would otherwise be very restricted.

Several hospitals in the United Kingdom have now, under the influence of the National Playing Fields Association, developed adventure playgrounds which have not only brought change to the mentally handicapped but have done a great deal to change attitudes and bring about an acceptance of hitherto not very well appreciated values of play and freedom to the mentally handicapped.

THE VALUE OF PLAY

The essence of all this is that mentally handicapped children can be – need to be – taught to play. They can be helped to discover the possibilities of toys. It is important to value the developmental level of the child in offering a play task. The play situation (learning situation) can be so arranged that the child need never fail, and also expanded to a level of adventure that allows the development of courage and the appreciation that life can be fun.

References

Adventure Playgrounds for Handicapped Children. (London: Handicapped Adventure Playground Association) (1978)

Guidelines for Playgroups with a Handicapped Child. (London: Pre-School Playgroup Association publication) (1978)

Perkins, E. A., Taylor, P. D. and Capie, A. C. M. (1976). *Helping the Retarded: A Systematic Behavioural Approach.* (Kidderminster: British Institute of Mental Health)

Wroe, B. (1979). *Organizing a Toy Library: A Description of the IMS Toy Library Service.* (Kidderminster: British Institute of Mental Health)

16

RESIDENTIAL PROVISIONS FOR THE MENTALLY HANDICAPPED

G. B. Simon

The mentally handicapped are at present accommodated in a variety of situations. In the past and at present the shortage, both in quantity and the range of residential facilities available in the community, has precluded much choice or selection but it is to be hoped that in the next 15 years placements will come to be made on the grounds of suitability rather than for administrative convenience.

THE FUTURE

From available information in the United Kingdom, a very approximate estimate of the present distribution of the severely mentally handicapped compared with a prediction of their likely placement in 1995 is shown in Table 16.1. These predictions are based on the recommendations of the White Paper (1971), current trends in care, progress over the past 5 years, and future plans, which have been agreed in principle but because of the financial restrictions will probably only materialize fully over the next 15 years.

Table 16.1 Present and predicted distribution of mentally handicapped

Location	Present distribution	Predicted distribution in 1995
Health Service provisions	27% (2% children; 25% adults)	11% (1% children; 10% adults)
At home	45% (20% children; 25% adults)	50% (25% children; (25% adults)
Other places in the community Foster-homes Group homes Hostels Lodgings Village communities	28%	39%

PATTERN OF RESIDENTIAL HEALTH SERVICES IN THE FUTURE

In most parts of Western Europe, the United Kingdom and the North American continent, the emphasis has shifted in spirit, if not in practice, in planning health and other residential services from large, frequently isolated institutions, to smaller establishments in the vicinity of the families they serve. There has been a marked reduction in the number of residents in most large hospitals in the past 10 years, and this is likely to continue. In the future, a hospital is unlikely to contain more than 200 beds. Although it is certain that many of the larger ones will continue to be needed for many years it has now become clear that their function is changing and will continue to do so. In their report *Helping the Mentally Handicapped in Hospital* (1979) the National Development Group provides details of the staffing, type of accommodation and services that are most appropriate in those that remain and the units which replace them.

Future residential health services for the mentally handicapped are likely to be provided in two forms: small local community units and a larger 'hospital' unit providing the more specialized services. The units forming the first part of this service are likely to consist of 16 to 24 beds sited conveniently close to the population they serve, which will vary from 60 000 to 120 000. The second part will be provided by larger units of no more than 200 beds and probably less, which support three or four community units and provide the specialist services referred to below, which it would not be possible to provide locally. Many of the hospitals of today already offer such services. Further explanations on the functions, role and services of the community unit and the hospitals are provided below, and more detailed descriptions can be obtained from Development Team reports, 1976–7 and 1978–9.

COMMUNITY UNITS AND COMMUNITY TEAMS

It is likely that some 40–50% of the health services required will be provided by community teams consisting of specialist medical, nursing, psychological and social work staff. These are likely to work from community units and be available for advice to schools, adult centres, hostels and other places caring for the mentally handicapped.

The intention is that the community unit should be flexible and able to provide an on-demand service, including relief to parents and others caring for mentally handicapped people at home, in hostels, schools and other places where experienced nursing or medical services are not always available.

SPECIALIZED SERVICES

Many of the more specialized services which cannot be provided at community units should be available at hospitals of less than 200 beds and serving populations of 250 000–500 000, depending on the geography of the area.

The predicted levels of provision in 1995 show a striking fall in the population of hospitals compared with the numbers in hospital today. This is accounted for partly by the fact that about half of the people at present in hospitals in England and Wales were admitted for very different reasons from those which should operate for hospital admissions in the future. Other factors which are likely to reduce the numbers in hospital are the effect of the services of specialist community teams and community units, coupled with an increase in the provisions and services of other agencies, e.g. social services, education and the voluntary associations.

The disabilities likely to require specialized services, not all of which will be possible at community units because of the staff required and the limited numbers likely to need them in the smaller population served by the community unit, are:

   (i) Behavioural difficulties requiring specialized assessment and programming.

  (ii) Severe behaviour and other problems requiring semi-secure accommodation with appropriate training.

 (iii) Special facilities for sensory handicaps – blind and deaf/blind mentally handicapped children and adults.

 (iv) Language- and speech-retarded mentally handicapped children and adults.

  (v) Mentally handicapped adults and children suffering from severe epilepsy.

 (vi) The physically disabled who require constant nursing and/or medical and paramedical services.

(vii) Major mental illness and other psychiatric disorders in the severely mentally handicapped.

SERVICES FOR THE MENTALLY HANDICAPPED LIVING AT HOME AND ELSEWHERE IN THE COMMUNITY

The majority of the *mildly* handicapped, and *some* of the severely mentally handicapped, will be very adequately provided for at special schools and through social services departments. From the experience of most professionals, however, it is clear that many *severely* handicapped and *some* mildly handicapped children and adults at home and elsewhere will require domiciliary specialist help if parents and others are to continue caring for them.

The tolerance of disability by parents, whether it be in the form of disturbed behaviour or incapacity of any sort, is usually far higher than is generally the case in most units apart from hospitals. Consequently, problems tend to be magnified; the only alternative when parents cannot cope, and need relief, is a health service unit, e.g. a community unit or a hospital. It will be essential for the members of the specialist mental handicap team to visit parents, assess the need and offer advice and support where necessary on management and training, to ensure that parents get the best out of their children. The chapter on 'Parents' Needs and How to Meet Them' makes it very clear that this service, coupled with relief when required, are the areas of greatest need.

References and Further Reading

National Development Group (1979). *Helping Mentally Handicapped People in Hospital.* (London: HMSO)

Reports of the Development Team for the Mentally Handicapped (1976–77 and 1978–79). (London: HMSO)

White Paper (1971). *Better Services for the Mentally Handicapped.* Command Paper 4683. (London: HMSO)

17

SEXUALITY AND THE MENTALLY HANDICAPPED

A. and M. Craft

In the past society's attitude towards the sexuality of mentally handicapped people has been inconsistent and negative. On the one hand, the mentally handicapped were thought to be asexual, lacking any sexual drive or need; on the other hand, mentally handicapped men were thought to be potentially sexually aggressive, and the women promiscuous (Tredgold and Soddy, 1963; Terman, 1916). Sexual information was withheld from them in an effort to keep them disinterested in sexual activity. Segregated colonies often gave preferential admission to women of child-bearing age (Cooke, 1973). Many of the old fears are still reflected today in the attitudes of parents and some care staff. In this chapter, we attempt to outline a positive approach to the sexuality of the mentally handicapped.

SEXUAL DEVELOPMENT

There are two aspects to human sexual development: first the biological growth and changes which take place during puberty; secondly, the psychosexual development which is a lifelong process. Do the mentally handicapped develop in ways which differ significantly from the normal population?

The Biological Aspect

About 30 in every 1000 general population are mildly mentally handicapped (IQ 51–70 on a standard IQ test) and can be expected to have normal physical and sexual characteristics. Three in every 1000 general population are severely mentally handicapped (IQ 0–50) and among these most develop normal physical and sexual characteristics, although there might be slight differences in timing. In Down's syndrome, which accounts for about one-third of all the severely mentally handicapped, the males tend to have smooth skins, do not need to shave until they are well into adulthood and although they can ejaculate, appear to be sterile. There is no known instance of a Down's syndrome man impregnating a woman. Down's syndrome females usually start to menstruate later than normal, but many do so eventually, although it may not be regular. In one study 58.8% ovulated (Salerno *et al.*, 1975); in another study 69.3% did so (Tricomi *et al.*, 1964).

Psychosexual Development

Psychosexual development is a complex and subtle process which begins at birth and continues throughout life. Usually it goes something like this. Babies find it comforting to be cuddled and by their reactions mothers are encouraged to prolong bodily contact. Small children are curious about their bodies and get satisfaction from touching the genital area. The attitude and behaviour of parents largely determines children's attitudes and behaviour. By the time schooling begins children have asked a lot of questions and begun role-playing and learning games with their peers ('mothers and fathers'). Before puberty most children associate mainly with their own sex and during puberty develop an interest in the opposite sex with much giggling and retreat to members of their own sex for exchanges of information and confidences. Adolescence is a state of very rapid growth – physical, psychological, intellectual and emotional. Some form of sexual experimentation is usually attempted, commonly heterosexual petting and masturbation. With maturity comes the establishment of stable social and sexual relationships, culminating in marriage and parenthood. This is an idealized version of the growing up process. We know from experience that for all sorts of reasons connected

256

with their upbringing, many people are not entirely at ease on matters of sex. They may feel guilty about sexual fantasies which they may have been taught to regard as 'dirty thoughts'; they worry about the adequacy of their sexual performance but never seek advice because they fear ridicule; they are embarrassed by the questions their children ask about sexual behaviour and are loath to talk about the sexual functions of parts of the body.

It is against this complex background we must look at what happens to the mentally handicapped child, who is born to a sheltered environment, and for whom complete independence may never be possible. Normal children usually share sexual experiences and information within peer groups, away from adult eyes and censorship; mentally handicapped children are closely supervised and also may not have the ability to communicate. Parents and care staff often find it easier to deny sexual experience to the handicapped child and over-react to displays of bodily curiosity, so that many mentally handicapped people have learned to be ashamed of certain parts of their bodies, to think of them as 'dirty', and any form of sexual activity as 'not nice'.

The mentally handicapped raised in institutions have additional difficulties when they reach puberty for the adults surrounding them are usually emotionally neutral to each other and there is no model upon which to base adult behaviour. Also, people's reactions to sexual behaviour differ and it is confusing when one member of the staff ignores solitary masturbation or homosexual activity, and another fiercely condemns it, whether it is done discreetly or openly.

Summary

Although the vast majority of the mentally handicapped are physically normal in development, their psychosexual growth may well be retarded because of the attitudes of those who care for them.

HEALTH AND SEX EDUCATION

Winifred Kempton (1972), one of the foremost writers in this field, reminds us of the special characteristics of mentally handicapped people which make health and sex education of *particular* importance:

1. They frequently over-respond to attention and give affection indiscriminately in return.
2. Their judgment may be poor, and their reasoning ability limited.
3. The mentally handicapped often do what is asked of them without question, and stand in danger of being used and exploited sexually.
4. Many do not have access to accurate information; their peers are usually equally ignorant.
5. They are likely to be confused and frightened by myths and half-truths because they find it difficult to distinguish between reality and unreality.

There are some questions always asked in discussions about sex education for the mentally handicapped:

Where sex is concerned, isn't it far safer to let sleeping dogs lie?
Surely what mentally handicapped people don't know can't hurt them?

The short answer is that ignorance is *not* bliss; rather it is a dangerous state. The question is never *whether* to teach mentally handicapped people about sex, but *who* does the teaching, and in *what form*? Learning about sex does not take place only in a formal way; most learning is acquired informally – from parental attitudes, from the way members of the family show affection, from talk and gossip, from television and the cinema, from advertisements, from watching how an elder brother behaves with his girlfriend. Mentally handicapped people have the same feelings and drives as the rest of the population. We do them a disservice if we neglect this part of social education, and do not give them the knowledge and understanding to withstand exploitation and enable them to satisfy their social and sexual needs without bringing them or others to grief.

Don't sex education programmes stimulate mentally handicapped people to experiment?

We have a folk saying about 'doing what comes naturally', and while there is plenty of evidence that withholding information about sexuality does *not* deter people from participating in sexual activity, there is no evidence that formal teaching stimulates normal or mentally handicapped children to sexual experiment. By giving children and adolescents a greater understanding of the changes taking place, both emotionally and physically, we could aid them to behave in a socially acceptable manner and avoid getting hurt.

Who Should Teach?

There is no 'obvious' choice; some parents would not want anyone but themselves to attempt it, others are only too happy for teachers or care staff to relieve them of what they find is an embarrassing task. What *is* important is that the person who tackles it is honest and direct, and at ease with the subject and the person or people being taught.

Topics to Cover

Mentally handicapped children and adolescents need to cover much the same ground as their normal peers (for a fuller discussion of topics see Craft and Craft, 1978). Each biological aspect must be set in its social context, for example:

Biological aspect
Puberty – physical changes in adolescence, emotional changes, increase of sexual interest and drive, start of menstruation, nocturnal emissions.

Social context
1. How does growing up change us?
2. Understanding ourselves and others – recognizing our own moods; how we signal what we are feeling?
3. Menstrual hygiene and care for girls. Knowledge of

259

menstruation for boys, in that they should know why girls are sometimes more 'touchy'.

4. Wet dreams – a boy will want reassurance that this is a normal occurrence.
5. Relationships with others of the same/opposite sex. Friends and acquaintances – do we behave in the same way to everyone? How do we decide how to behave? How do we try to make friends? What do we look for in a friend?
6. Girl-friends/boy-friends – what do you expect from them? What do they expect of you?
7. Public and private behaviour – is it sometimes different? Why?

Teaching Principles

1. Work either on a one-to-one basis, or with as small a group as possible (about four or five). Information exchanged in large groups is difficult to control; once members begin to talk readily they may listen hard to each other's misconceptions and fail to take in the teacher's correction. Don't have a very wide range of abilities in the group.
2. Remember this may be the first time the mentally handicapped person has been 'given permission' to ask about sexual matters. Be calm and unshockable.
3. It is helpful to have a good idea of how much individuals understand, and also of the main gaps in knowledge before starting. There is a manual available which can be used both beforehand to determine the extent of knowledge, and as a check on an individual's progress after a teaching programme (Fischer et al., 1973).
4. To teach we must communicate, it is pointless to talk about the 'penis' when the local and familiar slang expression is the 'dick' or 'cock'; so use language with which the group is familiar while introducing more socially acceptable terms for the various body parts.
5. Use plenty of visual aids. See Craft and Craft (1978) for a review of the audiovisual sources currently available.
6. Role-play can be an effective teaching tool, 'rehearsing'

situations and responses to them. For example, acting out behaviour on a date – the girl doesn't have to say 'yes' to everything.

7. Get them to repeat what they have learned, so that misunderstandings can be quickly corrected.

8. Teach at a realistic level. For example some mentally handicapped girls will only be able to grasp the hygienic aspects of menstruation; others will want to know more about the whys and wherefores; the brightest will be able to follow a simple explanation of its part in the reproductive process.

9. Listen carefully to the questions they ask and answer honestly.

10. Be flexible in timing and content. Just one slide on the screen or one picture in a book may involve enough information and discussion for a session.

EDUCATING PARENTS AND WORKING WITH THEM

Most parents have anxieties about the sexuality of their handicapped children. They do not always voice, or even acknowledge, their fears; instead they tend to over-protect. For example, they may not allow their son or daughter to go to a work training centre or social club; or they may insist that a member of the family always accompanies the handicapped person outside the home.

Professionals can do much to help parents by a matter-of-fact and practical approach. For instance, special school staff can hold parents' evenings for those with children approaching puberty, with advice on menstrual hygiene for the girls, and reassurance about nocturnal emissions (wet dreams) and masturbation for the boys. Or when the natural milestone of leaving school is reached, the work training centre staff may talk to parents in terms of young people growing up, wanting girl-friends or boy-friends, attending social clubs and dances.

Parents will often need practical help in deciding what and how to tell their child about sexual matters. There are a number of useful publications with illustrations, reviewed in Craft and Craft (1978); see also Shennan (1976).

Masturbation

Masturbation is a common problem for parents, because it frequently represents unmistakeable evidence that their son is showing an interest in sexual matters. (We discuss boys in this context as they are presented to clinics because of masturbation far more frequently than girls, but what follows holds good for both.)

First, parents should be reassured that masturbation is natural behaviour which is to be expected (Johnson, 1971). It is harmless and is very possibly beneficial where it is the only sexual outlet an individual has. Some mentally handicapped people may need guidance initially on how to masturbate to orgasm. For example, a severely subnormal young man may get very tense and disturbed by an erection because he has not discovered for himself the rhythmic stroking movements by which an orgasm can be achieved. For the handicapped at home fathers, or a male relative, are the best placed to teach the technique in privacy. Where this is not possible and mother requests professional help, what should be the response? The most important consideration is that the community nurse or social worker does not act in isolation. The same holds true for hospital or hostel care staff. A case conference should be held, which should include the nearest relative, recording the decision of the professionals involved that in their opinion it would be in the mentally handicapped client's interests to be taught how to masturbate, with the agreement of the nearest relative. This may seem an overly public approach to a very personal matter but professionals must safeguard themselves from complaint and possible prosecution for indecent assault, especially where the client is under 21 years of age, or is severely subnormal. We have reviewed the current legal position in detail elsewhere (Craft and Craft, 1978, ch.7).

Masturbation itself is not a problem but it becomes one when it is done in public – at school, on the bus, in the family living room. A professional asked by parents for help will need to explore several avenues.

1. Is there skin irritation present? or tight and ill-fitting clothing? This is not often the case but should be investigated as it is a possibility.
2. How does the adolescent spend his waking hours? Has he

enough interesting things to claim his time? Is he left sitting in front of the television set while the family do something else? Is he bored and lonely?

3. How do the family react if he masturbates in front of them? Is it the only time he becomes the centre of attention, and thus a very rewarding activity to him? Do his siblings giggle and make him feel he is making a joke? Does he do it to annoy his parents, perhaps after they have told him off about something?

4. Where does he usually masturbate? If it is in his bedroom or the bathroom, these should be recognized by the family as *private* not public areas, and his privacy respected.

Where masturbation persists in public, parents and day care staff should get together so that they adopt a uniform policy in the reshaping of the behaviour. Mentally handicapped people are quite capable of learning that masturbation, like toileting, is something to be done in private. Calmly removing the adolescent to the bedroom or bathroom at the first sign of such activity gradually makes clear what is expected. He can learn that pleasurable personal reward follows private masturbation; and that parental or care staff disapproval follows a public exhibition.

Adolescence is the time when there is much increase in sexual drive, and for some boys treatment by drugs may be advisable during a hyperactive phase. Specialist advice must be sought.

Parent Groups

Many parental anxieties get magnified out of proportion, and it is all too easy to see behaviour difficulties in terms of mental handicap, rather than the normal adolescent phase. This is especially true where the handicapped youngster is an only child. Informal discussion evenings for parents with a professional, who can talk knowledgeably about sexuality, can be a helpful means of sharing worries, comparing notes, and of offering and receiving advice and support.

HOSTEL AND HOSPITAL RESIDENTS

It is not always possible in hostels and hospitals to ensure that individuals have some privacy; this raises particular problems for staff and residents, as *all* behaviour is virtually public. Certain areas should be designated as private – bathroom, toilets and bedroom. Again the same principles apply – residents should have the opportunity to ask questions and learn about their bodies and emotions, with a framework of clear 'rules' of conduct. Residents should have the chance of having a say in the formulation of those rules at ward or hostel meetings.

Just as parents encourage some of their children's friendships, and discourage others, so might staff where they see a relationship developing which they feel is destructive. Discussions at staff meetings are essential in any unit because in talking about sexual behaviour the fears that people have about (and for) the mentally handicapped are aired and can be alleviated. Only when the idea of friendship, courtship and marriage is accepted in principle, can the staff meaningfully discuss whether a *particular* friendship is enriching a resident's life or not. For example a mentally handicapped woman may be more adept than staff at controlling her boy friend's aggressive outburst, not only because she stands no nonsense, but because her interest actually reduces his need to lose his temper. Or it may be that a mentally handicapped man takes advantage of a fellow resident, spending her money, smoking her cigarettes and eating her sweets, then ignoring her until her next pay day. In the first case staff might well decide that the friendship is mutually beneficial; in the second, that the girl is losing more than she is gaining.

Society seems to expect a higher standard of morality from mentally handicapped hostel and hospital residents than from other citizens. It should be remembered that in the eyes of the law the adult 'subnormal' person has the same rights as a normal citizen. He or she may marry, and if the male is over 21 he may enter into a private homosexual partnership with another adult (although not a 'severely subnormal') male. Legally staff have no right to prevent such actions. There is, however, an obligation on care staff to afford residents some protection from harm. In the context of sexuality this means sex education, pre- and post-marital counselling and making clear to males in particular the behaviour which is not permissible in public.

Some girl/boy friendships are 9-day wonders and cause more upset and worry to staff than to the two principals. Other relationships will grow and become serious. Quite early on, the couple might request marriage, and staff may well feel the pair have only a superficial understanding of what marriage entails. It may be helpful to have two clear stages, accepted by residents and staff alike as being reasonable. A couple saying they want to get engaged or married are told they must demonstrate the permanence of their feelings by 'going steady' for 3 months. The implications of this are usually well understood but should be further explained by staff, e.g. not going out with other girl/boy friends, helping each other, spending time together. The majority of relationships do not stand the test of time but then neither do many similar teenage friendships in the general population. All are learning experiences. In those which do, the couple may request engagement and marriage. A case conference with the couple, their families, and staff is held to discuss the future. A minimum engagement period of 6 months is usually set, giving time for premarital counselling, domestic training, finding accommodation and 'second thoughts'.

Conditions such as these are reasonable and allow time either for the pair to *learn for themselves* that they do not wish to make a life-long commitment or to enable everyone to plan a constructive future.

PERSONAL RELATIONSHIPS

Nearly all adolescents, normal or handicapped, present dilemmas and problems to those who care for them. But while everyone expects teenagers of normal intelligence to eventually become mature, independent and responsible, it is frequently not the expectation where mentally handicapped youngsters are concerned. Those who care for them are constantly faced with different aspects of a major dilemma. On the one hand, they want those in their care to develop their full potential and live enjoyable and happy lives; on the other, they see all too clearly the risks and unhappiness which might lie ahead if they allow them the freedom to make mistakes like the rest of society.

Some Do's and Don't's in Management

It is normal during adolescence to start having close friendships with members of the opposite sex. This is part of growing up. We have already discussed the need to prepare mentally handicapped youngsters for adulthood by sensitive sex education programmes. Parallel with this they need clear, reasonable and simply explained guidelines of behaviour, appropriate to their ability level.

What does all this mean in practice? First, that no mentally handicapped child should attain puberty without receiving some preparation for the changes that occur in growing up. Secondly, that parents and care staff must expect teenagers to develop friendships, and should encourage them to have as wide a social circle as possible. Most special schools and work training centres have weekly social clubs; like normal youngsters, the mentally handicapped teenager will also enjoy having friends in for an afternoon or evening, perhaps dancing to records or playing simple card and table games. If parents can withdraw to another room for a part of the time, so much the better. Rules of behaviour need to be clear; often mentally handicapped youngsters are uncertain about how loud the record player should be, how much they should eat, or what time they should go home.

When a mentally handicapped young person shows a special preference for a member of the opposite sex, parents or care staff are faced with a decision – should this be encouraged or not? If the feeling is mutual, there is much to be gained from such a friendship. Of course, *all* relationships carry with them an element of risk, but being hurt and let down by other people is as much part of being human as loving, caring and sharing and without these risks there remains little dignity in living. Again, the same principles apply and codes of conduct and the rules that apply will need to be clearly spelled out. Mentally handicapped youngsters usually do not have the finance, independence of movement, or social ability of their more normal peers. If a couple have no privacy and can only meet at home, or in the hostel dayroom when others are present then it is not realistic to tell them off for holding hands or cuddling in front of other people. Teenagers often talk in extremes, and if the girl says she loves and adores her boy-friend, adults should not over-react and think she is about to jump into bed with him – she is simply using the only word she knows to describe her excited and happy state.

BIRTH CONTROL METHODS AND THEIR INDICATION

Most parents will at some time wish to discuss contraception. An objection often raised to the use of contraception is that it only encourages the teenager to act irresponsibly. On the other hand, as with members of the general population, there is a likelihood that in some cases, and under some circumstances, intercourse may take place. Contraception is no more than a sensible precaution.

Some parents make the erroneous assumption that sterilization will not only end the reproductive capacity of their son or daughter, but also extinguish all sexual drive. This is not the case. Sterilization of minors is rarely indicated on medical grounds, and there are nearly always other satisfactory methods which may be employed and which are reversible. For girls who live at home or in hostels and hospitals, regularity in taking the pill can be ensured. For others not closely supervised an intra-uterine device, needing only periodic checkups, may be the most sensible method. Where engaged or married couples decide not to have children a male vasectomy is simple and effective. Professional advice is essential, and at a visit to the family doctor or family planning clinic, the options can be reviewed. There should also be locally available specialists familiar with the sexual development and needs of the mentally handicapped who can counsel both parents and professionals.

PARENTHOOD

Three aspects will be discussed here: the risk of handicap in children; fertility; and the parenting ability of mentally handicapped people.

Risk of Handicap in Children

At the beginning of this century, when modes of inheritance were less well understood, it was erroneously assumed that all mentally handicapped parents inevitably reproduced handicapped children, and to avoid this as far as possible, mentally handicapped people were prevented from mixing with the opposite sex. It has now been estimated that in any generation some 83% of the severely mentally handicapped children produced will have parents of normal intelligence (Reed and Anderson, 1973).

In a major study on mental handicap Reed and Reed (1965) surveyed 7778 children. In the 89 instances where both parents had IQs below 70 nearly 40% of the children were retarded (although the average IQ was 74). Where only one parent had an IQ below 70, 15% of the children were retarded (54% had IQs above 90). Of the 7035 children with neither parent mentally handicapped, 1% were retarded. Children's measured intelligence tends to revert towards the general population mean (Craft and Craft 1979a).

Fertility and the Size of the Family

We know that most mildly handicapped females and males have a normal biological capacity to reproduce but, if they are to care for their children adequately, then like the normal population they must be realistic about the size of their family.

Higgins *et al.* (1962) show clearly that there is no correlation between measured intelligence and family size. Mattinson's (1970) study revealed a lower birth rate for her mentally handicapped couples than in the general population. Our own Welsh survey indicated that mentally handicapped couples can be quite sensible and realistic in limiting the size of their families (Craft and Craft, 1979b). Only two of the 27 wives of childbearing age were not using contraceptive methods.

It is clear, therefore, that when advice and support is offered it can be of great benefit to mentally handicapped couples most of whom are quite capable of responding.

Adequacy of the Mentally Handicapped as Parents

This is by no means easy to assess. By what criteria should the adequacy of any parent be judged? What does seem certain is that the intelligence of the parents is only one of many factors which have a bearing on the quality of child care.

Other factors which will influence parenthood are similar to those which will affect any marriage and the attitudes of parents. Among the more important are marital harmony and stability; ill-health in either parent, physical or psychiatric; financial stress; number and spacing of pregnancies; and use of available support facilities.

The effects of the environment on development are now accepted. An interesting American project (Garber and Heber, 1977) attempted to prevent mental handicap arising from social and environmental deprivation by early intervention in a group considered to be at risk. Mothers participated in rehabilitative training and the infants had an intensive programme of sensory and language stimulation. At the age of 96 months one-third of the control children had IQs below 75 (WISC); by contrast the lowest IQ scores for the experimental children were two with 88. While the funds for such large-scale intervention are only rarely available, it should be possible to use existing resources through health visitors and social workers to aid mentally handicapped parents with their children.

Advice and Counselling on Parenthood

There are a number of questions which must be answered if meaningful advice is to be offered. For example, are one or both partners handicapped? If so, is the handicap a genetic one, with risks to offspring? Elsewhere in this book the genetics of mental handicap are discussed further. How old is the wife? If over 35 years do they realize that there is an increased risk of having a handicapped child? Are they likely to be able to cope with the complete dependence of a child over many years? What do they feel are the advantages and disadvantages of parenthood? Are these realistic? Many normal couples put off having a family until they have settled down together, and it is sensible to recommend this to a mentally handicapped couple. The aim of counselling is to clarify the often vague wish the couples have for a family and help them consider the practical implications.

MARRIAGE

One of the social revolutions of our times has been the advent of safe and readily available methods of birth control. For the first time in our social history it is possible to effectively separate marriage from parenthood. This has important implications for mentally handicapped people because marriage remains the socially acceptable and legitimate way of satisfying adult sexual ·and emotional needs.

How do mentally handicapped people cope with such a demanding relationship as marriage in which many 'normal' people 'fail'? In 1974, the authors carried out a survey within Wales of couples where one or both partners had been diagnosed mentally handicapped by a consultant. Our detailed findings are given elsewhere (Craft and Craft, 1978). We were sufficiently impressed with the care the majority of these couples gave each other, and their obvious subjective satisfaction with the married state, to extend the survey (Craft and Craft, 1979b). Through social services departments and health authorities, we located 45 couples where at least one of the pair had an IQ below 70. In fact, the 90 subjects were an extremely handicapped group – only 11 were of normal or dull normal intelligence and without disability. The other 79 subjects had at least one handicap, sometimes an additional two or three. So we were encountering people who would have required some form of help and support, whether single or married, and who were certainly at risk by any criteria. They were receiving a considerable amount of support from social workers.

While the nature of their problems had often altered after marriage, in nearly all instances we considered they had decreased in seriousness. It is significant that while approximately one in three marriages in Britain end in divorce, only one of our 45 couples had resorted to divorce.

Levels of personal satisfaction remained high; the partners had managed to offer each other a great deal of emotional and practical support, giving and getting much personal satisfaction in the process. From this study it would appear that with training, counselling and professional support, there could be many mentally handicapped people who might achieve the same satisfaction from life.

It is appropriate to end with the comment of one mentally handicapped couple, for they sum up the sentiments expressed by nearly all those interviewed:

WIFE: 'It's a lot better than when we were single. We are completely together and no-one can separate us. It's just great, you know.'

HUSBAND: 'Each can sort out the other's problems. Marriage is a wonderful life.'

CONCLUSION

It is unrealistic, and in the long run destructive, to assume that mentally handicapped people are without any sexual drives or feelings, and those who care for the mentally handicapped must accept their responsibilities in this area by thoughtful and sensitive teaching, training and counselling. At the very least mentally handicapped people should not be left in ignorance about their bodies and emotions, and thus in danger of being sexually exploited. We should, if we are to fulfil our responsibilities, create the supportive environment which will enable the mentally handicapped to develop their capacity for loving and caring relationships.

References:

Cooke, R. E. (1973). Ethics and law on behalf of the mentally retarded. In Haslam, R. H. A. (ed.) *The Pediatric Clinics of North America*, **20,** 259

Craft, M. and Craft, A. (1978). *Sex and the Mentally Handicapped.* (London: Routledge & Kegan Paul)

Craft, A. and Craft, M. (1979a). Personal relationships for the mentally handicapped. In Craft, M. (ed.). *Tredgold's Mental Retardation.* (London: Baillière Tindall)

Craft, A. and Craft, M. (1979b). *Handicapped Married Couples.* (London: Routledge & Kegan Paul)

Fischer, H. L., Krajicek, M. J. and Borthick, W. A. (1973). *Sex Education for the Developmentally Disabled: a guide for parents, teachers and professionals.* (London and Baltimore: University Park Press)

Garber, H. and Heber, F. R. (1977). The Milwaukee Project: indications of the effectiveness of early intervention in preventing mental retardation. In Mittler, P. (ed.) *Research to Practice in Mental Retardation,* vol. I, pp. 119–127 (London and Baltimore: University Park Press)

Higgins, J. V., Reed, E. W. and Reed S. C. (1962). Intelligence and family size: A paradox resolved. *Eugenics Quarterly,* **9,** 84

Johnson, W. R. (1971) Mental retardation and masturbation. In Rubin, I. and Kirkendall, L. A. (eds.) *Sex in the Childhood Years: Contemporary Views of Specialists in Childhood Sexuality.* (London: Fontana)

Kempton, W. (1972). *Guidelines for Planning a Training Course on Human Sexuality and the Retarded.* Philadelphia, Planned Parenthood Association of Southeastern Pennsylvania. (Available on loan, by post if necessary, from the library of the International Planned Parenthood Federation, 18–20 Lower Regent Street, London SW1Y 4PW)

Mattinson, J. (1970). *Marriage and Mental Handicap.* (Duckworth & Co.; Paperback edition published by Institute of Marital Studies, 1975).

Reed, S. C. and Anderson, V. E. (1973). Effects of changing sexuality on the gene pool. In de la Cruz, F. F. and LaVeck, G. D. (eds.) *Human Sexuality and the Mentally Retarded.* (London: Butterworth)

Reed, E. W. and Reed S. C. (1965). *Mental Retardation: A Family Study.* (Philadelphia: Saunders)

Salerno, L. J., Park, J. K. and Giannini, M. J. (1975). Reproductive capacity of the mentally retarded. *J. Reprod. Med.,* **14,** 123

Shennan, V. (1976). *Help your Child to Understand Sex.* (London: NSMHC)

Terman, L. M. (1916). *The Measurement of Intelligence.* (Boston: Houghton Mifflin Co.)

Tredgold, R. E. and Soddy, K. (1963) (eds.) *Tredgold's Textbook of Mental Deficiency.* (London: Baillière, Tindall and Cox)

Tricomi, V., Valenti, C. and Hall, J. E. (1964). Ovulatory pattern in Down's syndrome. *Am. J. Obstet. Gynecol.,* **89,** 651

18

THE LAW RELATING TO MENTAL HANDICAP AND TO THE MENTALLY HANDICAPPED OFFENDER

R. S. Bluglass

The present legislation relating to mentally handicapped patients can most easily be understood by reference to its historical origins.

In earlier times the law recognized only two forms of mental disorder, 'idiocy' and 'lunacy'. 'Idiots' had no understanding from birth and were thought to be incurable. 'Lunatics' developed their disorder at some later date and might improve or be cured. It was assumed that the mentally disordered required confinement against their will and normally this was arranged in appalling conditions and sometimes involved mechanical restraint. Originally 'idiots' were included with 'lunatics' in law but the Idiots Act of 1886 required separate arrangements for the confinement of 'idiots' and 'imbeciles' (a less-handicapped category).

The Mental Deficiency Acts of 1913 and 1927 derived from the recommendations of the Royal Commission on the Care and Control of the Feebleminded (1908) and they established local authority institutions specifically for handicapped patients. Mental deficiency was defined as 'a condition of arrested or incomplete development of mind (existing before the age of 18) whether arising from inherent causes or induced by disease or injury'. Four categories were defined: 'idiots', 'imbeciles', 'the feeble-minded' and 'moral defectives'. Under this legislation patients were usually admitted compulsorily, although institutions could in fact admit patients informally and after 1952 this was actively encouraged for short stays in hospital. However, all categories of 'mental defect' could only be admitted to designated hospitals.

The Mental Health Act of 1959 was the result of the deliberations of the Royal Commission on the Law relating to Mental Illness and Mental Deficiency (1954–57) (the Percy Commission) and it revolutionized the law by making informal admission the norm for all mentally disordered patients, as far as this is possible (including the mentally handicapped) and by allowing any hospital to take any kind of mentally disordered patient, if it could provide facilities for his care. Compulsory admission was restricted to certain types of patient. This change in the law resulted in a fresh outlook in the hospitals so that, by 1970, 97% of the severely subnormal and 89% of the subnormal were informal patients.

The Mental Health Act resulted in enormous advances in the care of the mentally disordered, in their status and in the way that the community regarded them, but in the years that followed the introduction of the new legislation there were further changes and development, in treatment and in outlook. In January 1975 the government decided to review the Act and in August 1976 published a discussion document which proposed a number of changes which might be incorporated in the law. After a period of discussion and debate a White Paper was published in September 1978 which described the amendments to the Mental Health Act 1959 which the last government intended to include in an amending Bill. The present Government is continuing this review.

THE DEFINITION OF 'MENTAL DISORDER'

The legal definition of mental disorder is given in Section 4 of the Mental Health Act 1959 as 'mental illness, arrested or incomplete development of mind, psychopathic disorder and any other disorder or disability of mind'. The Section sets out four sub-categories of mental disorder.

   (i)   mental illness
  (ii)   subnormality
 (iii)   severe subnormality
 (iv)   psychopathic disorder

The two degrees of mental subnormality are defined as follows:

Section 4 (2) 'severe subnormality' means a state of arrested or incomplete development of mind, which includes subnormality of intelligence, and is of such a nature or degree that the patient is incapable of living an independent life or of guarding himself against serious exploitation, or will be so incapable when of an age to do so.

Section 4 (3) 'subnormality' means a state of arrested or incomplete development of mind (not amounting to severe subnormality) which includes subnormality of intelligence and is of a nature or degree which requires or is susceptible to medical treatment or other special care or training of the patient.

It will be seen that the definition of 'severe subnormality' is based upon social functioning (the ability of the patient to cope in the community) while the definition of 'subnormality' is related to treatability. Although both definitions include subnormality of intelligence as one factor this is not described in terms of any specific IQ rating. This has been left to subsequent interpretation and avoids the possibility of relying upon an IQ assessment alone.

The last Government concluded in its proposals for change that the terms 'subnormality' and 'severe subnormality' cause offence and distress, and proposed that they should be replaced by the terms 'mental handicap' and 'severe mental handicap'.

It is also proposed that the two categories should be redefined so that the behavioural aspects of mental handicap will be adequately recognized. It is suggested that *mental handicap* will refer to *a state of arrested or incomplete development of mind which includes significant impairment of intelligence and social functioning. Severe mental handicap* would refer to *a state of arrested or incomplete development of mind which includes severe impairment of intelligence and social functioning.*

THE DEFINITION OF 'TREATMENT'

At the present time the definition of subnormality emphasizes the need for treatment. The Act defines treatment to include *care and training given under medical supervision.*

275

The White Paper acknowledges that this is a wide definition of treatment but thought that it may be too restrictive in relation to modern treatment programmes for the mentally handicapped. It is considered that a new definition of treatment is now required which would be more in line with today's perception of the needs of the mentally handicapped while still covering the treatment needs of other groups of the mentally disordered. The proposed new definition of treatment includes *'care, training, the use of habilitative techniques and medical nursing and other professional help'*.

ADMISSION TO HOSPITAL

Mentally handicapped patients, like patients suffering from other forms of mental disorder, can be admitted to hospital informally or compulsorily.

Informal Admission

Informal admission means that the patient can enter hospital without any formalities. It is assumed that he accepts his doctor's advice that he needs treatment and that he will normally stay in hospital until discharged. He may however leave hospital prematurely or decline to accept a particular form of treatment. The Act does not authorize staff to restrict an informal patient (for instance by locking him in a sideroom) or to detain him (for example in a locked ward). There is a duty under common law to offer treatment to patients and to prevent them coming to harm, so that the position of doctors and nurses can in some circumstances seem uncertain. An absence of objection to admission to hospital on the part of a patient who has the mental capacity to understand, at least in essence, what is being proposed, can be taken as implying consent. Those who refuse initially may respond to persuasion. Those who remain unwilling to enter hospital may have to be admitted under compulsory powers or remain in the community.

The law does not prevent mentally handicapped patients who develop mental illness from receiving all necessary care and treatment in a hospital which cares mainly for mentally handicapped patients. Despite this, practice varies in different parts of the country and the appropriate situation for the care of a particular patient is a matter of good practice and professional cooperation.

Compulsory Admission

The Mental Health Act 1959 provides short-term and longer-term powers for compulsory admission to and detention in hospital.

Short-term Powers

The short-term powers are:
1. Emergency admission to hospital under Section 29.
2. Admission for observation and assessment under Section 25.
3. Removal to a place of safety under Section 135.
4. Power of a constable to remove a person from a public place under Section 136.
5. Short-term detention of an informal patient already in hospital under Section 30.

These five classifications will now be examined in more detail.

1. Admission for observation in an emergency (Section 29)

Application: Can be made to the managers of the hospital by *any* relative or by a mental welfare officer*. The application must be supported by *one* doctor who need not be an approved doctor† (and in practice is usually the family doctor) and the patient must be admitted to hospital within 3 days from the date of the medical examination or the date of application (whichever is the earlier).

Grounds: The applicant and doctor must both indicate the urgent need for admission to avoid delay.

---

* A mental welfare officer is a social worker appointed by a social services department to perform the functions laid down in the Act. New proposals redefine the criteria for his appointment and role.

† A medical practitioner approved by a health authority as having special experience in the diagnosis or treatment of mental disorder. (Section 28, Mental Health Act, 1959.)

Duration: The power to detain the patient lasts for up to 72 hours from the time of admission.

Extension: The admission must be followed by a normal Section 25 or 26 recommendation within the 72 hour period or the patient must be discharged.

2. Admission for observation and assessment (Section 25)

Application: May be made by the patient's *nearest* relative or by a mental welfare officer who must have seen the patient personally within 14 days ending with the date of the application. It must be supported by recommendations by *two* doctors, one of whom must be an 'approved' doctor. The patient must be admitted within 14 days of the last medical examination.

Grounds: Must be that the patient is suffering from mental disorder of a nature or degree which warrants his detention in hospital under observation (with or without medical treatment) for at least a limited period in the interests of his own health or safety or for the protection of others.

Duration: The powers of detention last for up to 28 days.

Extension: A further application must be made to detain the patient, and this must not be only for further observation.

3. Removal to a place of safety (Section 135)

Application: A Mental Welfare Officer may if necessary give evidence on oath to a magistrate to obtain a warrant authorizing a constable to enter premises (if necessary by force), in order to remove a person thought to be mentally disordered to a place of safety so that his condition can be assessed and arrangements made for his care and treatment.

Grounds:
  (a) Where a mentally disordered person is being ill-treated, neglected, or not kept under proper control;
  (b) where he is unable to care for himself and is living alone;

(c) where he is subject to detention under the Act and is absent without leave and entry to premises has been, or is likely to be refused.

Duration: A patient may be detained in a 'place of safety'* for up to 72 hours.

Extension: A further application must be made under another section of the Act to detain the patient further.

4. Power of a constable to remove a person from a public place (Section 136)

Application: A police constable may remove a person from a public place to a 'place of safety' so that he can be examined by a doctor and be interviewed by a mental welfare officer, and any necessary arrangements made for his treatment and care.

Grounds: The patient appears to the constable to be suffering from mental disorder and to be in immediate need of care and control and it seems necessary to remove him in his own interests or for the care and protection of others.

Duration: Up to 72 hours.

Extension: He cannot be detained any longer unless further powers are invoked.

5. Detention of an informal patient who is already in hospital (Section 30)

Application: The responsible medical officer† can make a written report to the managers of the hospital‡ if he considers steps should be taken to invoke one of the compulsory powers to detain the patient in hospital.

* A 'place of safety' means residential accommodation provided by a local authority, a hospital defined in the Act, a police station, a mental nursing home or residential home for mentally disordered persons or any other suitable place the occupier of which is willing temporarily to receive the patient.

† The responsible medical officer is the medical practitioner in charge of the treatment of the patient (the consultant).

‡ The 'managers of the hospital' are the area health authority (or in the case of special hospitals the Secretary of State). Administrators act on the managers' behalf.

Grounds: It seems necessary in the patient's interests or for the protection of others to detain the patient compulsorily.

Duration: The patient may be detained for up to 3 days. (This may be changed to 72 hours by new legislation.)

Extension: One of the compulsory powers must be invoked to detain the patient further.

Longer-term Powers

The longer-term powers are:
1. admission to hospital for treatment (Section 26);
2. admission to hospital for treatment as a result of a hospital order made by a court (Section 60).

These will now be described in more detail.

1. Admission to hospital for treatment (Section 26)

Application: May be made by the patient's *nearest* relative or by a mental welfare officer, supported by two doctors (one of whom is an 'approved' doctor). The applicant must have seen the patient within 14 days and the patient must be admitted within 14 days of the last medical examination.

Grounds:
  (a) The patient must be agreed by the doctors to be suffering from a mental disorder which is:
    (i) mental illness or severe subnormality in the case of a patient of any age;
    (ii) psychopathic disorder or subnormality in the case of a patient who is under 21.
  (b) The disorder must be of a nature or degree which warrants the detention of the patient in hospital for treatment.

Duration: Up to 1 year.

Extension: The detention can be renewed for 1 further year and then for 2 years at a time by report to the managers of the responsible medical officer.

2. Hospital Order made by a court (Section 60)

Application: A court (Magistrates' or Crown Court) may make a hospital order in respect of certain criminal offences if the accused person has been found guilty and the court considers, taking all the circumstances into account, that this is the best way of dealing with the case.

Grounds:
   (a) The court must be satisfied on the evidence of two doctors (one an 'approved' doctor) that:
      (i) the patient is suffering from mental illness, psychopathic disorder, subnormality or severe subnormality; and
      (ii) the disorder is of a nature or degree which warrants the patient's detention in hospital for medical treatment; and
   (b) The court considers that this is the best method of disposal taking all the circumstances of the case into account.

Duration: This is for 1 year with similar powers to orders made under Section 26.

Renewal: The responsible medical officer must make a recommendation to the managers of the hospital within 2 months of the ending of the order if the power for detention is to be renewed, in the patient's own interests or for the protection of others. Subsequent renewals are required at 2-yearly intervals.

Special restrictions (Section 65)

The judge (in a Crown Court only) can (after hearing one doctor's oral evidence, but on his own decision) add a qualification that the patient cannot be given leave of absence, be transferred to another hospital or guardianship; can be called from leave at any time, and cannot apply to a Mental Health Review Tribunal *without the Home Secretary's consent**. The court is not required to receive the hospital's agreement to the application of a restriction order once a recommendation to

---

* Functions of Mental Health Review Tribunals; see p. 284.

make a hospital order has been put to a court. (However, new legislation would require the court to give advance notice to the hospital that a restriction order is being contemplated.) A restriction order can apply for a defined period of time or for an unlimited period (without limit of time). Proposed legislation would limit the use of a restriction order to cases when it is considered necessary 'to protect the public from serious harm'.

A Magistrates' Court may make a hospital order *without recording a conviction* (having received appropriate evidence) in the case of a person suffering from *mental illness* or *severe subnormality* if the court is satisfied that he is responsible for the act upon which the charge is based. The magistrates can also make a hospital order on a convicted offender, like the Crown Court, but if a restriction order seems necessary the case must be referred up to the Crown Court for consideration.

Special Hospitals

If the doctors making the medical recommendations think that the offender–patient is a person who requires treatment under conditions of special security on account of his dangerous, violent or criminal propensities, then the doctors can apply to the Secretary of State for Health and Social Services to provide accommodation in a special hospital. The Secretary of State is not obliged to accept everyone referred, but must be of the opinion that such conditions are necessary.

There are four special hospitals: Broadmoor, Rampton, Moss Side and Park Lane. Rampton and Moss Side take a slightly higher proportion of patients suffering from mental handicap or psychopathic disorder than do the other two hospitals.

Transfer to hospital of a patient serving a sentence of imprisonment (Section 72)

This part of the Mental Health Act authorizes the Secretary of State (Home Secretary) to issue a warrant to transfer a convicted prisoner to hospital. He must be satisfied:
(a) that the person suffers from mental illness, psychopathic disorder, subnormality or severe subnormality; and
(b) that the mental disorder is of a nature or degree which

warrants the detention of the patient in a hospital for medical treatment.

One of the two doctors making the recommendation must be an 'approved' doctor and the patient has similar status to a patient on a hospital order unless the Secretary of State has added restrictions as in Section 65 of the Act. The patient may be returned to prison if he recovers before the prison sentence expires. If still in hospital at that time his status becomes equivalent to that of a patient on a Section 60 Order. (Proposed legislation would change his legal status at the time at which he would be released from prison if he received full remission; after two-thirds of his sentence had been served.)

Transfer to hospital of a patient on remand in custody awaiting trial (Section 73)
Similarly a patient in custody awaiting trial can be transferred to hospital by the Secretary of State on receiving reports from two doctors that the patient suffers from mental illness or severe subnormality (but not psychopathic disorder or subnormality).

There are arrangements (Section 75) for the return of a Section 72 patient to prison and similarly for Section 73 patients (Section 76). The latter can be made the subject of a Section 60 order if his state would make it inadvisable for him to be returned to court.

GUARDIANSHIP ORDERS

A patient suffering from mental disorder can be placed under the guardianship of the local health authority or an approved individual if it is in the patient's interest or for the protection of others. The application is similar to a Section 26, but is made to the health authority within 14 days of the last examination. For psychopathic disorder and subnormality the age limits (see above) apply. The guardian has the same powers as a father of the patient, as if the patient was under the age of 14 years (Sections 33 and 44).

OTHER MATTERS

Mental Health Review Tribunals

Mental Health Review Tribunals are established by the Mental Health Act to review the need to continue to detain patients on compulsory orders. Patients detained under Sections 26 and 60 may apply for a review within the period of 6 months from the date of the order or from the day that the patient reaches his 16th birthday. Patients on Section 65 (restriction) orders must be referred by the Home Secretary. The Mental Health Review Tribunal may discharge from detention or guardianship.

The government is considering new legislation for automatic reviews of detained patients, conditional discharge and new Rules of Procedure for the Tribunals.

Duration of detention (under Section 26 and Section 60) and guardianship

The duration of these orders is limited by Section 43 to 1 year, but can be renewed for a further year and then for periods of 2 years, if an appropriate recommendation is made to the managers of the hospital and accepted. (Proposed legislation would halve these time-periods to renewal after 6 months and then at annual intervals.) Those on restriction orders can only be granted leave of absence or be discharged by the Home Secretary on the recommendation of the responsible medical officer with or without conditions regarding place of residence, supervision by a social worker, attendance at a clinic or other requirements.

Relatives

Relatives have certain rights of discharge for Section 26 patients, but this can be overruled by a recommendation from the responsible medical officer (if accepted by the managers).

Offences against Patients

Ill treatment of patients (Section 126) and sexual intercourse with patients (Sections 127 and 128) are offences which can lead to a conviction. Sexual intercourse with individuals known to be severely mentally handicapped is an offence even if they are not patients.

New Legislation

The government's recommendations will alter time-periods relating to detention and review of detention, and also aim to strengthen the rights of patients in hospital. New forms of hospital order are proposed which will give a court power (on receiving recommendations) to remand a mentally handicapped offender to hospital for assessment. Powers to make an interim hospital order to give a trial of treatment are also contemplated.

CRIMINAL RESPONSIBILITY AND MENTAL HANDICAP

Fitness to Plead

Mental handicap may lead to a finding that a person accused of a criminal offence is *unfit to plead,* if he cannot understand the nature of the charge against him; cannot distinguish between the meaning of 'guilty' and 'not guilty'; cannot challenge a juror, instruct counsel or follow the proceedings in court. He would be sent to a hospital nominated by the Home Secretary and his status will be equivalent to a person detained under Section 65 of the Mental Health Act.

Criminal Responsibility

A person charged with any criminal offence may plead *not guilty by reason of insanity* if at the time of committing the offence he did not know what he was doing or did not know that it was wrong in law, as a result of a defect of reason due to disease of the mind. These rules were established by the famous M'Naghten case. Only four or five people in England and Wales make a successful plea of this kind each year, so that this aspect of the law is virtually in disuse. A successful plea would lead to detention in a hospital nominated by the Home Secretary as if on a Section 65 (restriction) order.

New legislation recommended by the Butler Committee on Mentally Abnormal Offenders redefines this part of the law and if accepted by Parliament will widen its use.

Diminished responsibility

In murder cases, only, a mentally handicapped person (like others who are mentally disordered) may be able to plead that at the time of the act or omission (that led to the victim's death) he was suffering from 'such abnormality of mind as would substantially impair his mental responsibility'. A jury can accept or reject this on the evidence and if accepted the patient would be guilty not of murder, but of manslaughter. This is an offence allowing any appropriate disposal by the judge including a hospital order or probation order with a requirement of treatment if recommended.

Mitigating features

For other offences, it may be put to the court that the patient's mental state or limitations might be borne in mind in deciding the best disposal or limiting the sentence. Recommendations for a medical disposal of the case are usually given serious consideration and are accepted in most cases (Bluglass, 1979).

Probation with a requirement of psychiatric treatment

Probation supervision can be ordered by a court if the patient agrees to co-operate with the requirements of the order (Powers of Criminal Courts Act 1973). This may be helpful in the management of patients who are not severely mentally handicapped. A requirement of treatment as an inpatient or outpatient can be added on the recommendation of one 'approved' doctor for any period up to 3 years duration.

THE MENTALLY HANDICAPPED OFFENDER

In the past 'mental deficiency' was considered one of the most important factors in the aetiology of criminal behaviour, but the Mental Deficiency Acts of 1913 and 1927 substantially reduced the proportion of mentally handicapped appearing before the courts and being accommodated in prisons. The greater the degree of mental handicap the more likely it will be that an offence will be detected as a result of poor organization and clumsy execution. The severely subnormal is easily recognized and will usually be found unfit to plead; if tried, he is unlikely to be considered responsible for his actions and in either case will receive a medical disposal, usually to hospital.

Those of subnormal or borderline intelligence are more likely to be in trouble as a result of impulsive behaviour, a sudden episode of anger, limited tolerance to alchohol or sexual frustration than as a consequence of the failure of a carefully planned and premeditated crime. Sometimes the mentally handicapped are exploited by others to take risks and take part in illegal behaviour. Some in a childlike way do not understand, or fail to appreciate, the implications of their actions and may find themselves the subject of a criminal charge.

Brain damage and epilepsy are rarely the sole cause of delinquent behaviour but may be associated with other factors such as emotional deprivation, disordered or broken homes and mental handicap; the problems which may underlie delinquency in persons who are not mentally handicapped.

Chromosome abnormalities occurring in persons of limited intelligence have also been associated with delinquency, particularly the XXY chromosome complement and XYY syndrome (see Chapter 3). These cases are of special interest but probably represent no more than a further predisposing factor in the delinquency of a small group of patients.

Types of offence

The limitations and particular characteristics of mentally handicapped offenders are associated with a tendency to commit specific offences. Walker (1968) compared the indictable (serious offences) committed by all male offenders aged 17 or more, and dealt with by English courts in 1961, and the offences of the 305 males of similar age, who were committed to hospital by criminal courts as being subnormal or severely subnormal. The percentage of subnormal offenders dealt with for sexual offences was six times

as high as the percentage of all offenders. The mentally handicapped patient is more likely to be sexually uninhibited, less well-
controlled and more likely to find comfort in the company of
children. At the same time society's prohibitions on sexual expression are more difficult for the mentally handicapped to comprehend.

Mentally handicapped patients are not more likely to commit
offences of violence than other individuals, and the majority of
their offences, like those committed by offenders generally, are
mainly property offences such as theft, criminal damage or
occasionally arson. When committed by mentally handicapped
offenders these offences are more often trivial and they are less
skilfully carried out.

Care of Mentally Handicapped Offenders

The majority of mentally handicapped offenders can be cared for
in ordinary hospitals for the mentally handicapped without difficulty. There are however a small but important number who
require special conditions with more staff and a higher degree of
security than is normally available. The government has initiated a
policy of providing 'regional secure units' for each Regional Health
Authority to care for the mentally ill and some mentally handicapped patients (Bluglass 1978; Oxford Regional Health Authority, 1978). In some regions special units for the severely mentally
handicapped are being planned.

Mentally handicapped patients of dangerous, violent or criminal
propensities on restricted hospital orders are accommodated at
Rampton or Moss Side Hospitals.

LEGISLATION IN SCOTLAND

Scotland has separate mental health legislation (the Mental Health
(Scotland) Act 1960). Mental disorder is defined as 'mental illness
or mental deficiency however caused or manifested' and 'mental
deficiency' is defined no further.

Compulsory Admission

The Mental Health (Scotland) Act, 1960 provides *short-term* and

288

longer-term powers for compulsory admission to and detention in hospital. The legal authority for admission is the Sheriff Court.

Short-term Powers

The short-term powers are:
1. emergency admission to hospital under Section 31;
2. removal to a place of safety under Section 103;
3. power of a constable to remove a person from a public place under Section 104;
4. detention of a patient already in hospital under Section 32.

These four powers are now examined in more detail.

1. Emergency admission to hospital (Section 31)

Application: Can be made to the sheriff by any medical practitioner on the day of the medical examination. The recommendation should be supported by the consent of a relative or mental health officer, where practicable. The patient must be admitted within 3 days.

Grounds: Admission is urgently necessary by reason of mental disorder.

Duration: The powers of detention last for a period not exceeding 7 days.

Extension: The patient must be discharged, may remain in hospital as an informal patient or a further recommendation under Section 31 may be made.

2. Removal to a place of safety under Section 103

Application: A mental health officer or medical commissioner may give evidence on oath to a justice of the peace to obtain a warrant authorizing a constable to enter premises (if necessary by force) in order to remove a person suffering from mental disorder to a place of safety with a view to making an application or emergency recommendation or other arrangements for his treatment or care.

Grounds:
  (a) where a mentally disordered person has been or is being ill-treated, neglected or not kept under proper control;
  (b) where he is unable to care for himself or is living alone or uncared for;
  (c) where he is subject to detention under the Act and is absent without leave and entry to premises has been or is likely to be refused.
A medical practitioner should accompany the constable in the case of (a) and (b). In the case of (c) a medical practitioner and any other person authorized to take the patient may be present.

Duration: A patient may be detained at a place of safety* for a period not exceeding 72 hours.

Extension: The patient must be discharged unless another order is invoked.

3. Power of a constable to remove a person from a public place (Section 104)

The Scottish legislation is similar to Section 136 of the English Act except that an interview with a social worker is not required. A responsible person residing with the patient and the nearest relative must be informed of the patient's removal 'without delay'.

4. Detention of patients already in hospital (Section 32)

An application for admission or an emergency recommendation may be made with respect to patients already in hospital and the patient will then be treated as if admitted to hospital on the date on which the application or recommendation was made.

Longer-term Powers

The longer-term powers are:
1.   admission to hospital for treatment (Section 24);

---

* A 'place of safety' under the Scottish Act means a hospital, a residential home for persons suffering from mental disorder or any other suitable place the occupier of which is willing temporarily to receive the patient; but shall not include a police station unless by reason of emergency no other place is available.

2. admission to hospital for treatment as a result of a Hospital Order made by a court (Section 55).
These two powers are now examined in more detail.

1. Admission to hospital for treatment (Section 24)

Application: May be made by the *nearest* relative or an authorized social worker (who can over-rule the relative but must then inform him of his right of appeal to the Sheriff). The application must be supported by two doctors, one of whom is an 'approved doctor'*, but they may only examine the patient together when no objection has been made by the patient or his nearest relative. The application must be submitted to the Sheriff within seven days of the medical examination. The Sheriff may make any enquiries he wishes. The patient may be admitted within seven days from the date upon which the Sheriff gives approval.

Grounds: The doctors must agree on the form of mental disorder from which the patient suffers which may be:
  (i) mental illness or mental deficiency or both;
  (ii) and that the disorder requires or is susceptible to medical treatment and is of a nature or degree which warrants the patient's admission to hospital,
  (iii) and that the interests of the health or safety of the patient or the protection of others cannot be otherwise secured;
  (iv) a patient over the age of 21 cannot be made the subject of an application for admission (or be received into guardianship) if he is suffering *either* from mental deficiency such that he is capable of living an independent life and guarding himself against serious exploitation *or* mental illness which is manifested only by abnormally aggressive or seriously irresponsible conduct.

Duration: Twenty-eight days or 1 year.

Renewal: The detention is renewable for a further year and is then renewable at 2-yearly intervals.

* Approved under Section 27 of the Scottish Act.

2. Hospital Order made by a Court (Section 55)

Applications: A court (High Court of Justiciary or Sheriff Court) may make a hospital order in respect of an offender found guilty of an offence punishable by imprisonment, to detain him in a specified hospital or to place him under the guardianship of a local authority.

Grounds: The court must be satisfied on the written or oral evidence of two medical practitioners (one of them an 'approved doctor'):
 (i) that the patient is suffering from mental disorder of a nature or degree which would warrant his admission to hospital under Section 24 (see above). The age limitations do not apply to the two disorders indicated in Section 24:
 (ii) that the court considers, taking all considerations into account, that a hospital order is the most suitable method of dealing with the case.

Duration: The responsible medical officer must review the case between 21 and 28 days after the order is made and again after an interval of 1 year and then at 2-yearly intervals unless the patient is discharged. The patient is otherwise detained as if under a Section 24.

Special restrictions
A judge in the High Court or Sheriff Court may add restrictions relating to the discharge of a patient on a hospital order if he considers it necessary for the protection of the public. One 'approved' doctor must give oral evidence. The effect of the restriction is similar to the English restriction order, but only the Secretary of State for Scotland has the power to discharge the patient (absolutely or conditionally) and the equivalent of the right of the patient in England to request a Mental Health Review Tribunal to review his case rests with the Mental Welfare Commission. All patients in Scotland can complain to the Commission concerning any matter relating to treatment or detention and they are usually interviewed personally by the Commissioners. Restrictions may be with or without a time limit and the Secretary of State may remove them, when the

patient's status becomes that of a patient on an ordinary hospital order.

A Sheriff Court may (in the case of a person charged under summary procedure*) make a hospital order without recording a conviction if the court is satisfied that the accused is responsible for the offence with which he is charged.

State Hospital

The court may specify that the offender patient should be sent to the state hospital at Carstairs (Scottish equivalent of a special hospital) after hearing evidence that special security is needed.

Transfer to hospital of prisoners

There are similar arrangements in Scotland for the transfer to hospital of patients serving a period of imprisonment on the direction of the Scottish Secretary of State (Section 66).

GUARDIANSHIP ORDERS IN SCOTLAND

There are similar arrangements in Scotland for Guardianship Orders under Section 25 of the Mental Health (Scotland) Act, although for 'psychopathic disorder' (undefined) and minor mental handicap the age limit of 25 does not apply. Although guardianship in Scotland was based on a tradition of 'boarding out' the mentally handicapped on crofts and farms before the 1960 Act, as in England its use has declined.

MENTAL WELFARE COMMISSION

The Scottish Mental Welfare Commission has no equivalent in England. It consists of between seven and eleven Commissioners appointed by the Crown and its task is to safeguard the welfare and interests of individual patients (informal and detained). It has no responsibility for the running of psychiatric hospitals. At least one of the Commissioners must be a woman, one a lawyer and three must be doctors. The Commission must exercise a protective function in respect of persons who may by reason of mental

---

* Summary procedure is equivalent to trial in a Magistrates' Court in England.

disorder be incapable of protecting themselves or their interests.

The Commissioners may discharge any patient except a restricted hospital order patient, can advise informal patients about their legal rights, can inquire into ill-treatment or deficiency in care of treatment and may consider complaints. The Commission has a duty regularly to visit detained patients and patients under guardianship. The Commission's powers apply also to patients in the community. It has an important function to protect patients' property and financial interests by making investigations and suggesting appropriate action. Members may see hospital records, compel the attendance of witnesses, take evidence on oath and have a duty to discharge wrongfully detained patients and to advise the Secretary of State of their findings.

CRIMINAL RESPONSIBILITY AND MENTAL HANDICAP IN SCOTLAND

Insane in Bar of Trial

A person who is so mentally handicapped or mentally ill that he is unable to defend himself properly may, in Scotland, be found 'insane in bar of trial'. The issue is usually raised by the defence and may be decided by the judge or be left to the trial jury. If the case is a serious (indictable) offence before a High Court or Sheriff Court the judge must order the patient to be detained in the state hospital (or elsewhere if there are special reasons). The order is equivalent to a hospital order with restrictions of unlimited duration. If the case is a less serious one being dealt with under the summary procedure, the court can make a hospital order with or without restrictions. A higher proportion of offenders are found insane in bar of trial in Scotland than are found 'unfit to plead' in England, and they tend to stay in hospital longer than those found fit to plead (Chiswick, 1978).

Criminal Responsibility

An accused person may plead insanity in the higher courts. To do so it must be shown that at the time of the act or omission there existed some mental defect by which his reason was overpowered and he was thereby rendered incapable of exerting his reason to control his conduct and reactions. The test is wider than in England and includes the possibility that a person may not understand what is happening even though he is aware of the nature of the act and that it is wrong.

Diminished Responsibility

The concept of diminished responsibility was introduced into the common law of Scotland in 1867. A charge of murder may be reduced to culpable homicide (which does not carry the fixed penalty of life imprisonment) if it is shown that the accused suffered at the time of the act or omission from a state of mind bordering on insanity, and if the court accepts that it was of sufficient degree to diminish responsibility. Unlike the situation in England the prosecution can bring the lesser charge without waiting for the defence to raise the matter of diminished responsibility. It is probable that the concept of diminished responsibility is more severely applied in Scotland than England.

Probation Orders with a Condition of Psychiatric Treatment

Although there is no probation service in Scotland a court may make a probation order with a condition of treatment but the condition can only be made for 1 year although the probation supervision can continue for 3 years. The supervision is carried out by a local authority social worker.

MANAGEMENT OF PROPERTY AND THE MENTALLY HANDICAPPED

The Court of Protection (Part VIII, Mental Health Act 1959)

Some patients suffer from such a degree of mental handicap that they are incapable of managing their own affairs. The Court of Protection's principal officers are the Master and Deputy Master and judges nominated by the Lord Chancellor, and their function is to 'do or secure the doing of all such things as appear necessary or expedient' for the maintenance or other benefit of the patient or his family, or for providing for other people or purposes for which the patient might have been expected to provide were he not disordered, or for otherwise administering his affairs (Section 102, Mental Health Act 1959). The Act contains a list of some of the actions that the court may do on a patient's behalf. Before accepting a patient within its jurisdiction the court must be satisfied on medical evidence that the patient is incapable by reason of mental disorder of managing and administering his property and affairs.

The judge may act in an emergency if necessary (Section 104, Mental Health Act 1959).

Wills

In order to make a will, a patient must be capable of understanding the nature of the business with which he is engaged, recollecting the property he means to dispose of and the persons who are the possible beneficiaries, and indicating the manner in which it is to be distributed between them. A doctor, nurse or other person caring for the patient should always seek an independent medical opinion about the patient's testamentary capacity should he wish to make a will to avoid any future dispute and suggestion of undue influence having been made.

Mentally handicapped patients may be incapable of making a will and if necessary the Court of Protection can make a will on the patient's behalf.

PROTECTION OF THE PATIENT'S PROPERTY IN SCOTLAND

In Scotland the Mental Welfare Commission has a duty to ensure that the property of all mentally disordered patients is not exposed to loss or damage; and it has powers of investigation regarding patients' financial affairs.

There is no equivalent of the English Court of Protection. Instead, if two doctors certify a patient's incapacity the Court of Session can appoint a *curator bonis* to manage the property and affairs (usually a solicitor or accountant). This is usually applicable in relation to estate worth £1000 or more. For the administration of smaller amounts the hospital authority can be empowered to act for the patient. There are rules governing these arrangements.

THE MENTALLY HANDICAPPED AND OTHER LEGAL MATTERS

Marriage

A marriage will be void (as if it had not taken place) if either party did not give proper consent to it because of 'unsoundness of mind' (Matrimonial Causes Act 1973). This would only apply if at the time of the ceremony one of the parties could not understand the nature of the contract being entered into and 'appropriate its basic responsibilities'.

A marriage will also be void if at the time of the marriage either party, although capable of giving valid consent, was suffering (whether continuously or intermittently) from mental disorder within the meaning of the Mental Health Act. This must be 'of such a kind or to such an extent as to be unfitted for marriage' (i.e. incapable of living in a married state and carrying out the ordinary duties and obligations of marriage). The proceedings must be brought within 3 years of the marriage.

Divorce

The sole ground for divorce is now that the marriage has irretrievably broken down in one of five specified ways (see Matrimonial Causes Act 1973). Mental disorder may contribute to any one of these.

Matrimonial and Care Proceedings Before Magistrates

Magistrates' courts may make decisions about maintenance or custody of children where a 'matrimonial offence' is proved (for example, adultery, desertion, persistent cruelty and wilful neglect). If the parents are incapable of looking after their children properly (because of the parents' mental disorder, for instance) the children may go into the care of the local authority voluntarily or as a result of care proceedings (Section I, Children and Young Persons Act 1969).

Driving

An applicant for a driving licence must inform the authorities if he suffers from any disorder for which he is compulsorily detained, if he is receiving in-patient treatment informally, if he suffers from severe subnormality for which he is under guardianship, is receiving any form of local authority care or suffers from any form of disorder for which his property is in the hands of a receiver. The Department may refuse a licence although there is a right of appeal.

Income, Employment and Social Security Benefits

The rights of the mentally handicapped in relation to security of employment, contracts of employment and business matters are outside the scope of this chapter. For details about these important matters and for a description of the arrangements for assisting patients and their families through social security benefits (including contributory and non-contributory basic scheme benefits, industrial injuries benefits and supplementary benefits) the reader is referred to *Mental Health,* by Brenda Hoggett (London: Sweet & Maxwell)

Further Reading

Bluglass, R. (1978). Regional secure units and interim security for psychiatric patients. *Br. Med. J.*, **1**, 489

Bluglass, R. (1979). The psychiatric court report. *Medicine, Science and the Law*, **19**, 121

Chiswick, D. (1978). Insanity in bar of trial in Scotland. *Br. J. Psychiatry*, **132**, 598

Chiswick, D. (1979). Operating the Mental Health Acts. *Br. J. Hosp. Med.*, **21**, 167

Gostin, L. O. (1975 and 1977). *A Human Condition*, vols I and II. (London: National Association of Mental Health)

Hoggett, B. (1976). *Mental Health*. (London: Sweet & Maxwell)

Mental Health Act 1959. (London: HMSO)

Mental Health (Scotland) Act 1960. (London: HMSO)

Oxford Regional Health Authority (1978). *A special care unit for mentally handicapped patients*. Report of a Working Group. (Oxford Regional Health Authority)

Report of the Committee on Mentally Abnormal Offenders (The Butler Report). Cmnd. 6244. (London: HMSO)

Review of the Mental Health Act 1959. Cmnd. 7320. (London: HMSO)

Walker, N. D. (1968). *Crime and Insanity in England*, vol. 1 (Edinburgh: Edinburgh University Press)

Walker, N. D. and McCabe, S. (1973). *Crime and Insanity in England*, vol. 2. (Edinburgh: Edinburgh University Press)

INDEX